W9-BFB-215

# Yoga
## on the
# Ball

# Yoga
## on the
## Ball

Enhance Your
Yoga Practice Using
the Exercise Ball

*Carol Mitchell*

Healing Arts Press
Rochester, Vermont

Healing Arts Press
One Park Street
Rochester, Vermont 05767
www.InnerTraditions.com

Healing Arts Press is a division of Inner Traditions International

Copyright © 2003 Carol Mitchell

All rights reserved. No part of this book may be reproduced or utilized in any form or by any means, electronic or mechanical, including photocopying, recording, or by any information storage and retrieval system, without permission in writing from the publisher.

*Note to the reader: This book is intended as an informational guide. The remedies, approaches, and techniques described herein are meant to supplement, and not to be a substitute for, professional medical care or treatment. They should not be used to treat a serious ailment without prior consultation with a qualified health care professional.*

**Library of Congress Cataloging-in-Publication Data**

Mitchell, Carol.
Yoga on the ball : enhance your yoga practice using the exercise ball / Carol Mitchell.
p. cm.
ISBN 0-89281-999-5
1. Yoga. 2. Swiss exercise balls. I. Title.
RA781.7.M547 2003
613.7'046—dc21
2003008566

Printed and bound in the United States at Capital City Press

10   9   8   7   6   5   4   3   2   1

Text design by Cindy Sutherland
Text layout by Virginia Scott Bowman
This book was typeset in Goudy with Avant Garde as the display typeface

# Contents

# Introduction

*Yoga:*
*Tradition and Innovation*

Some revolutions begin quietly.

A little more than a century ago a learned man from India made his way to the United States to participate in a pan-religious conference convened in conjunction with the Chicago World's Fair. The Parliament of Religions, held in 1893 in Chicago, hosted representatives from a multitude of cultures and faiths, including Jains, Sikhs, Baha'is, Mormons, and Rastafarians. Native Americans, Catholics, Protestants, and evangelicals were also present. Representing the Hindu faith was Swami Vivekananda, a young and inspiring monk with a gift for eloquence and a burning passion to serve humankind.

Translated literally, the word *yoga,* derived from the Sanskrit *yug,* means "to yoke," to join or unite. Simply put, yoga is a set of practices meant to harmonize the various aspects of our being—body, mind, and spirit—by "yoking" these fragments of ourselves into an integrated whole, a being grounded in individual and universal consciousness.

Historians estimate that yoga is at least five thousand years old and may have been developed as much as tens of thousands of years ago. There is evidence to suggest that a system similar to yoga was practiced in the ancient Mayan, Indian, and Tibetan cultures. Various yogalike postures are depicted on scrolls found in Tibet that date back to approximately 40,000 B.C.E.

References in the Rig-Veda, India's oldest text on mysticism and religion, confirm that yoga was practiced in the Indus Valley as early as 3000 B.C.E. The people of the Indus Valley were ultimately conquered by invading tribes from Russia and Central Asia. The conquering tribes, known as the Aryans, spoke Vedic, the precursor of classical Sanskrit. Over time Vedic society and religion absorbed many of the cultural and spiritual practices present in the Indus Valley at the time of its invasion. Around the second century B.C.E. the sage and Sanskrit scholar Patanjali composed the primary text of yoga, the Yoga Sutra, distilling and codifying the far more ancient wisdom of this physical and spiritual practice.

Yoga made its way to many Middle Eastern countries during the Muslim invasions, around C.E. 1200. It wasn't until the late 1800s that yoga concepts found their way to Western civilization as a result of Western scholars translating the ancient Indian texts. Eastern philosophy began permeating some Western intellectual circles of the day, evidenced especially in the works of transcendentalist writers such as Henry David Thoreau and Ralph Waldo Emerson.

Soon Hindu holy men, or *swamis,* began to make visits to Britain and the United States to share yoga philosophy and practices. Swami Vivekananda won over Western audiences in his 1893 visit, a notable feat, because at the time many in the West viewed India as a land of infidels. Vivekananda awed people everywhere he spoke. When he spoke at the Parliament of Nations the deafening applause lasted for three full minutes. Vivekananda's eloquent speeches created a curiosity and respect for Eastern religions in the West.

In 1920, a few decades following Vivekananda's debut, the International Congress of Religious Liberals hosted Paramahansa Yogananda, another Indian spiritual leader. As this accomplished yogi and spiritual master traveled throughout the United States sharing his knowledge he interested thousands of Westerners in yoga philosophy. Paramahansa Yogananda moved to California in 1925 and founded a yoga center that he named the Self-Realization Fellowship; that center is still in operation today. In 1946 Yogananda authored the story of his spiritual journey. His *Autobiography of a Yogi* further accelerated the West's curiosity about this body of spiritual teachings from the East.

Interest in yoga's physical postures—the branch of yoga referred to as hatha yoga—increased in the 1940s when Indra Devi, a European woman who lived in India and studied yoga with Sri T. Krishnamacharya, began to teach yoga to movie stars in her studio in Hollywood. Soon Americans and Europeans started visiting India in search of a deep spiritual experience and greater understanding of the life enrichment that yoga offered. Hatha yoga was introduced to millions through Richard Hittleman's *Yoga for Health* television show, which premiered in Los Angeles in 1961, and Lilias Folan's nationally syndicated television show, *Lilias! Yoga and You!*, which ran from 1972 to 1992 and became the yoga practice guide for millions more in the West. Thousands of people began to practice yoga and meditation when their interest was sparked after the Beatles' trip to India in 1968.

By the 1970s the field was fertile for Hindu yogis to begin teaching yoga in the West. B. K. S. Iyengar, another student of Sri T. Krishnamacharya, began traveling to the West in the 1950s and by the early 1970s had followers all over North America and Europe. There was a thirst among people in the West to learn as much as they could about this ancient practice. Yoga was here to stay.

Flash forward to the present. The April 2001 issue of *Time Magazine* reported that fifteen million Americans have had some exposure to hatha yoga, and a recent survey by *Yoga Journal* revealed that one in thirteen Americans had practiced or were interested in trying hatha yoga. Yoga classes are presently being offered at health clubs, spas, YMCAs, community centers, and private studios. The Chicago Bulls and the Miami Dolphins practice yoga; so do Jane Fonda, Christy Turlington, Madonna, Sting, and Kareem Abdul Jabbar, their celebrity greatly raising the public profile of yoga in recent years. The Royal Canadian Mounted Police and even the fire department in Los Altos, California, use yoga for physical conditioning and stretching of the body. It is not hard to imagine that hatha yoga is perhaps the most widely practiced exercise system in the West today.

## Tradition and Innovation

Yoga's introduction to the West came about through the vision of a few pioneering souls willing to step respectfully outside of tradition in order to further the spiritual development and humanity of the world's citizens. As the first monk to leave India in order to teach the timeless message of the yogic scriptures to the rest of the world, Vivekananda broke with tradition; he lost his caste standing as a result. When he was criticized for teaching the Vedic wisdom to foreigners Swami Vivekananda explained that the lover of God has no caste restriction. Vivekananda's fearless actions destroyed old conventions, opening the way for many spiritual teachers from the East to come westward.

Sri T. Krishnamacharya, born in India in 1888, a few years before Vivekananda traveled to the West, is acknowledged by many as being the grandfather of modern hatha yoga. Born in 1888 into a family that practiced yoga, Krishnamacharya studied yoga for many years with distinguished masters. Most of his study revolved around the practice of ayurvedic medicine and the therapeutic use of yoga postures (*asanas*) and breathing practices (*pranayama*). (Ayurveda incorporates the use of herbs, purgatives, and oils to help balance the body's energy system.) Krishnamacharya became an ayurvedic doctor and prescribed yoga to his patients, customizing the asana work to meet each patient's individual needs. Krishnamacharya would revolutionize the teaching of yoga by encouraging those who studied under him to "teach what is inside of you, not as it applies to yourself but as it applies to the other." He believed that yoga should be adapted to fit the student rather than the student adapting to "fit" yoga. Krishnamacharya refused to standardize his practice and teaching methodology, thus making yoga accessible to a broader range of people.

Krishnamacharya's philosophy helped shape the development of the hatha yoga culture in the West. His strength laid in his ability to bridge his vast knowledge of yoga and the body with his keen insights about changing values and practices of modern-day life; Krishnamacharya's genius manifested in his ability help others adapt yoga to fit their own needs, interests, and lifestyles. Krishnamacharya's principles and teaching style empowered his students to develop forms of yoga distinctly their own.

Several offshoots of Krishnamacharya's teaching are today's most popular forms of hatha yoga known to the West. A look at a few manifestations of Krishnamacharya's wide influence will be telling.

B. K. S. Iyengar, after whom Iyengar yoga is named, was a student of Krishnamacharya. The Iyengar style of yoga utilizes props such as straps, blocks, bolsters, and other tools designed to make postures more accessible for the beginning student, or for those dealing with physical constraints and conditions that would not otherwise let them practice yoga. Iyengar yoga involves fewer poses than other systems of yoga but places great emphasis on perfecting alignment. Iyengar yoga is practiced widely in the West today.

Pattabhi Jois, also a student of Krishnamacharya, developed ashtanga yoga as his translation of Krishnamacharya's work. This physically challenging style of yoga is comprised of increasingly difficult postural sequences accompanied by the use of bhandas (body "locks") and breathwork to produce strong internal heat for purifying muscles and organs, expelling toxins, and releasing beneficial hormones. The posture sequences are to be followed precisely to be in alignment with Pattabhi Jois' teachings.

Another evolution of Sri T. Krishnamacharya's philosophies is viniyoga, a yoga style developed by Krishnamacharya's son and student, T. K. V. Desikachar. Viniyoga focuses on the movement of the body through the initiation of the breath and involves creating an individualized practice for a student incorporating breathwork, postures, chanting, and meditation.

Each of these yoga styles—Iyengar, ashtanga, and viniyoga—had their origins in the teachings of Sri T. Krishnamacharya, an important innovator who provided a model for developing a style of yoga practice that fit the present-day needs of his students at the time. Many yoga students in the West followed

Krishnamacharya's lead—once hatha yoga was introduced in the West some interesting offshoots began to develop.

Inspired by the teachings of Paramahansa Yogananda, J. Donald Waters created ananda yoga, a system that encourages deep release and relaxation into yogic postures while using affirmations to heighten awareness, all in preparation for meditation.

Various forms of "power yoga" have evolved as Western adaptations of ashtanga yoga. This athletic form of yoga, consisting of breathwork and choreographed sequences of advanced postures, is particularly attractive to athletes and those who are already highly conditioned.

Several modern-day yoga styles incorporate dance as an important element of practice. A fluid, dancelike version of hatha yoga was created by Kali Ray, director of the Tri-Yoga Center in Santa Cruz, California. This meditative form of movement consists of a flowing sequence of precise postures paired with breathwork and meditation. Danskinetics, created by Ken Scott, a longtime student of Yogi Amrit Desai, combines the natural flow of Kripalu yoga with dance. Rasa yoga evolved from Danskinetics. Rasa yoga combines yoga, music, and free-form dance that builds to an ecstatic release.

As an antidote to the pressures of twenty-first century life, Judith Lasater's restorative yoga brings about deep relaxation in the entire body by practicing postures with the support of pillows, blankets, bolsters, and straps. Donna Farhi incorporates developmental movement principles as fundamental preparation for a yoga practice that is in supportive relationship with gravity. Psychology and classical asanas are joined in Michael Lee's Phoenix Rising Yoga Therapy, a style of yoga that incorporates sixteen poses designed to promote physical balance, spiritual awareness, and mental and psychological healing.

It is within this lineage of tradition and innovation that I introduce a new adaptation of the five-thousand-year-old spiritual and physical discipline of yoga. The exercise ball, like yoga, has a long and varied history. Used for decades by physical therapists, the exercise ball (or Swiss ball, as it is traditionally called), has recently been "discovered" by a wider fitness population. Exercise balls are indispensable tools for keeping the mind engaged in the activity at hand, the unstable surface keeping you ever attentive to the shifting needs of the body for balance at any given moment. Balls are important tools for supporting the musculoskeletal system during rehabilitation from an injury and for enhancing sport performance.

It is known that balls were used for fitness and stimulation as far back as Galen's time. In the second century Galen, an influential Greek philosopher and physician, wrote that exercising with a ball "can stir the enthusiast or the slacker, can exercise the lower portions of the body or the upper." He also noted that "the best athletics of all are those that not only exercise the body but are able to please the spirit."

Yoga on the Ball provides a unique mind-body training opportunity made possible only by marrying the properties of the exercise ball with the attentions and intentions inherent in the practice of yoga. As a surface made soft or strong by the amount of air inside, the ball can be used either as a base of support for working with difficult yoga postures or as a tool for intensifying the stretch in a targeted area of the body. Many people find that the ball aids them in sinking more deeply into a satisfying yoga stretch and helps them execute yoga strengthening and balancing asanas that they were previously unable to achieve.

Welcome to this exploration of a new yoga—steeped in tradition, updated for our times, using a simple prop to help us achieve depth in our practice.

Enjoy your journey.

Namaste.

# 1
# Yoga and the Ball— A Dynamic Duet

My personal journey with yoga began when I was a university student in the late 1970s. I had been told that yoga could help a person manage stress and I figured I was going to have a lot of it ahead of me in school, so I began seeking opportunities to become acquainted with the discipline. My first exposure to yoga was in a religious studies class; I remember being utterly taken aback by the seeming intricacy and extensiveness of this ancient system. I was particularly drawn to raja yoga, the path of yoga tht works with the mind to keep thoughts and actions focused in a spiritual direction, and even though I had never heard philosophical views like these before, I felt completely at home with them. They touched something deep and familiar in me. I was very appreciative of the meditation skills I was learning and knew that yoga was going to be part of my lifelong study.

I took the opportunity to study yoga academically every chance I got. Blessed to have professors who shared the personal benefits they gleaned from yoga, my own curiosity continued to be peaked. I took every available academic course and recreational class in yoga studies available to me. By the time I completed my degree I had studied extensively (at the novice's level) the spiritual tenets of yoga and had practiced various forms of hatha yoga, including Iyengar, viniyoga, and kundalini yoga.

In university I studied health sciences and psychology; those disciplines in tandem with yoga gave me a valuable foundation for my first "real" job as a crisis counselor in a shelter for battered women. In my role as counselor and confidante I shared some of the meditation skills that had become treasured tools to me. It's important to be able to cultivate a haven deep within yourself in which you can rest and rejuvenate. Yoga had helped me to develop that sense of equanimity, and I found that, in the support of the crisis center, the clients I worked with there were at least open to trying to make that haven for themselves. Time and again in positions of employment in various mental health settings I was blessed with supervisors who supported my desire to share the yoga tools I had developed for myself with the people we were serving.

Several years after my graduation from university I became certified as a fitness instructor, a personal trainer, and ultimately as a medical exercise specialist. It was through that course of study that I began to see fitness and yoga as a marriage of great potential. As part of my studies I began updating many of the traditional yoga postures to reflect current exercise science. Many classic yoga postures push students past what we now know to be a safe range of motion. Following the inspiration of Sri T. Krishnamacharya, acknowledged by many as the grandfather of modern yoga, I began adapting yoga postures to meet the needs of the student rather than manipulating the student to fit the practice of yoga.

It wasn't until I was pregnant with my first child that I began adapting yoga postures to the exercise ball. I was working toward my brown belt in muay Thai boxing at the time, and my obstetrician and I agreed that it would be best if I hung up my boxing gloves for a while. I had been keeping up with my yoga practice throughout my pregnancy, yet as my pregnancy progressed I found that some of the deep lunges were irritating my knees. And because my center of gravity was changing I found some of my favorite postures difficult to execute without losing balance. I was also missing the variety that I enjoyed in my martial arts class. I needed something to help me stay in shape but I also needed it to feel manageable and safe, and fun!

Adapting yoga to the exercise ball was the answer. Most people recognize that both yoga and ballwork tone muscle. What is especially unique about Yoga on the Ball is the fact that by rolling in and out of the asanas we work more of our muscles and hit on the muscle fibers from varying angles while negotiating the pose. We can also change the intensity of the exercise by modifying our body's positioning on the ball. In exploring how to adapt yoga to the exercise ball I realized that this was the way I would be able to maintain muscle tone and fitness during my pregnancy and could use the ball as an important support for balance, as well as for consciously challenging my balance.

Another benefit I realized in my early adaptation of yoga to the ball was the way it worked my core musculature and challenged the endurance capacity of the stabilizing muscles along my spine. The core musculature consists of three deep muscles of the trunk: the transverse abdominis, the quadratus lumborum, and the multifidus. A strong, stable core is essential to back health, protecting the spine by preventing excess rotating, sliding, or bending of the vertebrae and subsequent compression of the vertebral discs. Without a stable core everyday movements, a fall or an unexpected jarring, or even sitting with poor posture can leave you vulnerable to injury.

Moving through yoga asanas on the ball, or even simply maintaining an easy seated pose on the ball, forces the stabilizing musculature of the spine to have to work in order to keep you from falling off the ball. Increased incidence of sedentary living in our society contributes to a lack of tone in these important muscles. Movements that challenge the stabilizing muscles along the spine can be micro in nature but macro in effect—every time these muscles are called into play it results not only in a more aesthetically pleasing, toned set of abdominals but also in a more solid foundation that will help align and protect the back.

Many fitness programs emphasize the large muscle groups but neglect to train the smaller stabilizing muscles. We have already talked about the stabilizing muscles in the core area and the back; actually there are stabilizing muscles throughout the body. Wherever they are located the stabilizers protect you from injury by surrounding the joint and securing the joint in place. Think of the orchestration necessary to bend and straighten the knee. Small stabilizing muscles at the knee joint, such as the vastus medialis obliquus, secure the patella, the bony structure of the knee, while the hamstrings flex the joint and the quadriceps extend the joint. Or consider the stabilization work that goes on at the shoulder joint when you lift your arm overhead. The small rotator cuff muscles (supraspinatus, infraspinatus, teres minor, and subscapularis) must all work together to hold the humerus, the long bone of the arm, in the joint when you reach your arm overhead.

These are big names, and big jobs, for very little, very important muscles. Training on an unstable surface, such as an exercise ball, conditions these stabilizing muscles. When you sit on the ball and raise one leg off the floor in Tree pose you rely on your core as well as on the stabilizing muscles of your lower leg to keep you balanced. Reaching your arms overhead in Prayer Breath you rely on the rotator cuff muscles to secure the arm in place at the joint so you can lift your arm overhead and flex and extend the shoulder joint.

Balance is also improved by executing yoga asanas on the ball. Every time the body is required to perform its balancing function the vestibular system is called upon. This miraculous, complex system, housed in both inner ears, is made up of a labyrinth of chambers and canals filled with water. When your head moves, voluntarily or otherwise, the fluid moves too, which causes tiny hairs in the canal to bend. The dance of these hairs triggers a firing of nerve impulses, which in turn cause the brain to direct adjustments to the parts of the body needed to keep you from falling off the ball. This constant orchestration between the nervous system, the vestibular system, and the muscles keeps you balanced as you sit in or roll into a yoga asana.

Imagine being able to maintain your balance when your dog tugs at his leash and breaks into a full run without so much as a second's notice, never mind staying balanced in the athlete's work of running, jumping, crouching, cutting, and changing directions in rapid-fire fashion. You need good balance and strong stabilizers in order to keep from being injured, especially when a load is added to the movement—that load might be the dog pulling on his leash, the groceries you lift out of your trunk, or the basketball you dribble down the court.

Improved posture is another benefit of the Yoga on the Ball program. In compiling this book great care has been taken to select yoga asanas that strengthen some muscles and stretch others in order to create the muscle balance in the body that is necessary to help the body maintain ideal alignment.

All of these benefits designate Yoga on the Ball as a functional workout. Functional workouts stretch some muscles and strengthen others. They help develop balance and coordination. They improve core stability and foster efficiency in the stabilizer muscles. A functional workout is one that includes elements that will enhance performance, whether in sport or everyday activity, not only by training the "power" muscles but also by working the systems that prevent you from becoming injured. It is great to be strong, but you must be able to stabilize your body properly for the strength to be optimally employed. If you are an athlete and you do not train your stabilizers you will not have the edge that other athletes who've trained for stability have.

Another element of a functional workout is incorporating methods that change the intensity of the workout. We can change the intensity of a Yoga on the Ball asana simply by shifting the relationship of the joints or by placing more or less of the body on the ball. With Yoga on the Ball you can build a beginner-level practice or an intense advanced sculpting workout, or you can choose to simply enjoy gentle, soothing stretches, all the while building endurance through a workout that is eminently applicable to your daily life.

A final note on the benefits of pairing yoga asanas with the exercise ball:

working on the exercise ball can make the practice of yoga safer for some populations. When I was pregnant my knees hurt continually. My ligaments were loose due to the hormone relaxin circulating through my body and preventing the ligaments in my knees from being as stable as they could be to hold the knee joint in place properly. It seemed I was constantly twisting my knees, and the pain was ever present. The ball provided support for my body weight so that I could perform a half lunge, which allowed me to continue practicing Sun Salutation (although I did not sink so deeply into the asanas). Had I not altered my practice by using the ball I could have caused damage to my knees.

A client of mine who had fairly new hip replacements found it just too difficult to hold certain yoga asanas, because she did not have the muscle strength to support the hip joint in the early stages of her post-rehabilitation. With the use of the ball partially supporting her body weight she felt safer and was able to execute previously challenging asanas, postures that were of great benefit to her hips and thighs.

Because the ball can be easily positioned to give you cushioned support where you need it, those who suffer from chronic pain conditions such as fibromyalgia or arthritis may find that they are not as sore after this form of exercise. The ball also allows you to rest in a chairlike fashion if fatigue becomes overwhelming. Many people recovering from an injury or dealing with chronic pain concerns will find a welcome friend in the ball.

In the chapters to come you will be introduced step-by-step to the principles that inform a Yoga on the Ball practice and the asanas that will help you devise your own Yoga on the Ball session.

Chapter 2 starts you on your journey with instruction in yogic breathing and exercises to help you relax and anchor your mind in present-moment awareness. These are handy tools to put in your stress management kit. You may find that these tools can make you more effective at work, giving you an edge by helping you to think more clearly and creatively. You might find that breathing well helps to calm you, and that communication inside your treasured relationships, your relations with family and friends, improves as a result. Many of my students have told me that working with the breath has given them a passageway to serene spiritual adventures. For many breathwork is a tool that facilitates communion with the Divine, however you define that numinous force.

Finding comfort in your body through postural explorations is the topic that is discussed in chapter 3. The spinal alignment explorations in this chapter foster postural awareness in everyday living—good posture contributes to spinal health and improved overall functioning of the musculoskeletal system. In this chapter you will also be introduced to the body's core musculature—important muscles in the trunk, including the transverse abdominis, that work to protect the spine when the body is in motion. For many people the transverse abdominis is a greatly underused muscle that, when awakened, not only gives one a more stable base to move from but also provides the added benefit of an aesthetic, toned trunk. These explorations will adequately prepare the body for yoga asana practice; a thorough understanding of the material presented in this chapter can change the way you sit, stand, and move. You will want to take your time learning and assimilating these postural awareness concepts into your life and your practice.

In chapter 4 we discuss the importance of customizing a warm-up to fit the activity you will be engaging in. All too often many of us do not give a second thought to the preparation that our muscles, minds, and central nervous systems need in order to prepare for undertaking a physical activity, whether sport, hobby, or task. Adequate preparation for physical activity is absolutely essential. In this chapter you will be learning the Yoga on the Ball version of the Sun Salutation, a yoga-specific warm-up consisting of a flowing sequence of basic postures. This is the activity-specific warm-up that I recommend you use prior to every Yoga on the Ball session; you can use the Yoga on the Ball Sun Salutation for cardiovascular conditioning too. Chapter 4 also addresses the importance of using your abdominal muscles throughout your Yoga on the Ball practice. You will be introduced to the concept of a yoga "lock" and to uddiyana bhanda—truly one of yoga's ancient and best secrets! The simple act of working with this lock during your Yoga on the Ball practice will tone your abdomen and strengthen your core musculature, stabilizing and toning your trunk and making your movement more efficient. A stable core also helps protect the back from strain and injury.

Striking the balance between strength and flexibility is the theme of chapter 5. This chapter introduces classic yoga postures adapted to the exercise ball. Readers are encouraged to analyze their lifestyle habits and current levels of strength and flexibility in order to personalize the Yoga on the Ball practice for targeting the body's needs. This chapter also addresses sequencing the yoga practice to achieve maximum benefit for the body.

Chapter 6 addresses the body's need for strong balancing skills. Good balance translates into greater skill in your fitness or sport activity and a reduced possibility of injury in unexpected situations, such as preventing a fall on an icy path or easily regaining center when a dog tugs suddenly at its leash. The postures in this chapter provide opportunities to slow down and breathe into the moment so that you can not only improve balance but improve your stress management skills as well.

The chapter outlining the advanced postures will help experienced practitioners of yoga and ballwork to discover their edge. It is imperative that you have a good command of the asanas in chapters 5 and 6 before moving on to the advanced work. These postures are unique and fun; most revolve around developing a strong, stable core and long, lean muscles. Be meticulous in following the cuing and moving slowly through each step.

The chapter 8 asanas will help you to relax and rejuvenate. If you need stress management tools this is the chapter for you. Ending a Yoga on the Ball practice session with restorative poses is a good way to lock in the benefits of your asana practice—when you relax deeply at the end of an asana practice your nervous system "grooves" the memory of the muscle releases for future reference. You may also find that the relaxation and breathing exercises in this chapter provide you with a ritualized, workable format for relaxing into meditation or prayer, setting the stage for a more serene way of living. No doubt you will find that practicing these postures on a regular basis will reward you with more peaceful and relaxed moments in your life. So take the time to experiment with these postures and determine which are your personal favorites. Every one of us is individualized in our interests, preferences, and sense of pleasure even when it comes to relaxation and rejuvenation.

Chapter 9, "Putting It All Together," provides you with three practice sessions—a basic practice, an advanced practice, and a restorative practice—to help you begin integrating Yoga on the Ball into your everyday life.

## Choosing Your Exercise Ball

There are a number of exercise balls on the market, and most certainly there is variation in terms of quality. When I first began to work with the exercise ball I purchased one at a local department store. After only a few short weeks of having the ball it burst while I was gently bouncing on it. I was lucky that I did not hurt myself. This incident led me to do my homework in researching the various exercise balls available to the consumer.

Had I known what to look for at the time I could have purchased a quality ball for the same amount of money that I spent on a cheap one. I recommend that you acquire an anti-burst ball that is pressure tested to one thousand pounds and has a nonskid surface. The most comfortable ball I have found to work with is the Fitball. This ball is anti-burst and will support several hundred pounds of pressure. It also has a specially treated surface that makes it less likely to slip on the floor and you to slip off it. The balls are available in black, white, lavender, and multicolored. Most of my students prefer the pastel lavender ball, maybe for its relaxing color. Information on how to order a Fitball can be found on page 182.

Recommendations about the specific diameter (size) of ball a person should use for physical exercise varies depending on the teacher and the activity. The larger the ball the more difficult it is to control. A general guideline for use of the exercise ball is this: when you are sitting squarely on the center top of your ball you want your knees to be in line with your hips and your hips and knees both bent at a 90-degree angle. You don't want your thigh bones to slope precipitously downward from the hips (the ball is too big) or to be higher than the hips (the ball is too small). For people 5' to 5'8" tall a 55-centimeter ball usually suffices. For those 5'8" to 6'2" a 65-centimeter ball will generally work best.

When you first begin working with the ball you will likely feel as if you have more control over the ball when it is smaller. After you have had some experience with the exercise ball and with practicing yoga asanas you may find that you want a slightly larger ball to increase the challenge. You will want to experiment somewhat with the inflation level of the ball as well. A slightly deflated ball is more easily controlled and is less likely to drift than a fully inflated ball. People who are new to ballwork often commence working with a slightly deflated ball and then move on to a greater inflation level as they progress in their practice. Most important in this equation is that you determine what is most comfortable for you and what works best for your practice goals. The ball you work with should provide you with the correct level of challenge in your practice.

Many ball companies sell a small hand pump specifically designed to inflate exercise balls. Bicycle pumps are slow to inflate a ball; air compressors are forceful and require vigilance so that the ball is not overinflated (which is dangerous—"anti-burst" is only applicable within a ball's given maximum diameter). If you acquire a small hand pump when you purchase your ball you may find you are more likely to tote the ball along with you on vacation, or to use it as an alternative desk chair at work when you need.

Those who sit at a desk for long hours may find a good friend in the ball. The ball's inherent instability requires the body to make continual microadjustments to keep the spine erect. This constant small shifting keeps the muscles of the back and pelvis from fatiguing, as is the case when you sit in a chair for too long. You can also roll on the ball to change the points where your body makes contact with the ball's surface, which decreases the likelihood of experiencing the tension or local burning sensations in the muscles that often accompanies sitting for an extended period of time. To use a ball as a chair you need to determine the size that will best fit the desk you sit at. Many people find a softer, slightly deflated ball to be preferable to a taut, fully inflated ball when using the ball for a desk chair.

Let's begin our exploration of Yoga on the Ball now at the point where each of us began this human life—the breath.

# 2
# The Body and the Breath

Yoga on the Ball practice is built on the foundation of the breath. Breathing fuels every system in the body, each full breath stoking the cells with a copious supply of life-giving oxygen. By focusing our attention on the wavelike, ever constant ebb and flow of the breath we help to center ourselves, strengthening perception of our surroundings and responding with calmness and integrity to the energies of the moment. Anchored in the present we receive what is to be lived in each moment; we are not swallowed up by chaotic thoughts or recurring whirlwinds of emotion.

The practice of *pranayama*—regulating life energy by consciously controlling the breath—is a valuable tool developed by the ancient yogis, who sought not only to connect with their highest self but also to become one with all of humankind and nature. The yogis' ultimate goal was to create balance and harmony of mind, body, and spirit. Many modern-day relaxation, breath-therapy, and breath-training programs for athletes are based on these ancient yogic teachings of the East.

Every time we take a breath we help to create balance both in our bodies and in the world around us. The act of respiration creates balance outside of the body by providing much needed carbon dioxide to the environment, which is then converted to food for plants. Within the body, breathing creates balance by continuously supplying the cells with fresh oxygen, which helps

16

the cells release their excess carbon dioxide. Without this exchange cells rapidly die from oxygen depletion and a buildup of waste products.

Yogic breathing involves strong, steady, movement of the diaphragm, a thick umbrella-shaped muscle that separates the chest from the abdomen. The diaphragm originates at the sternum, travels down the sides and back of the body to the lower ribs, and is anchored in the back to the vertebrae that make up the upper part of the lower spine. On the inhale oxygen is drawn in through the trachea to the lungs; in this inhalation phase the diaphragm contracts downward toward the belly. The abdomen expands as the diaphragm presses downward and breath fills the lungs. On the exhale the diaphragm relaxes and recedes upward, compressing the lungs, and air is therefore expelled. The abdomen gently contracts to its "resting" state. This up-and-down diaphragmatic action massages the internal organs, keeping them well nourished with fresh blood.

We come into this world fully equipped for taking deep, diaphragmatic breaths. Through infancy most people breathe freely and easily from the diaphragm. However, by adulthood most people who do not practice some sort of Eastern-based body or meditation discipline develop shallow breathing patterns. When we breathe shallowly the oxygen tends to collect in the top part of the lungs, where there is less blood for the oxygen to mix with; both the heart and the lungs have to work harder to extract the necessary oxygen and circulate it throughout the body to fuel the body's processes. The rapid loss of carbon dioxide through short, shallow breaths leaves a person in a state of chronic hyperventilation.

How do we evolve into chest breathers? Certainly posture has a great deal to do with shallow breathing. I find that most people who come to me for a fitness consultation require some sort of postural retraining. Most of us spend a great deal of time each week sitting in vehicles and working at desks or on computers. If we are not vigilant about our posture it is all too easy to slump when we are involved in these tasks. If your shoulders are rolled forward and you have succumbed to a forward-thrusting head position, you cannot possibly take a full breath into your lungs.

Clothing can also place restrictions on our breathing. How often have you felt that you just could not take a deep breath when you were wearing tight pants or a belt? It is vitally important to put some thought into how you dress if you want to encourage healthy breathing patterns on a day-to-day basis. Shallow chest breathing also commonly develops as a response to stress. A remark I often hear from students in my yoga class is that they know they are under stress but didn't recognize the stress manifesting in their breathing patterns.

The ancient yogis believed that every human being who comes into this life is given a certain number of breaths, and that if you breathe quickly and shallowly you will die sooner than someone who breathes slowly. Chest breathers tend to take approximately sixteen to twenty respirations per minute whereas diaphragmatic breathers respire six to eight times per minute.

Many people report being astonished by the difference in the way they feel the first time they experience breathing from the diaphragm. Diaphragmatic breathing helps balance the sympathetic and parasympathetic nervous systems, aspects of the nervous system responsible (respectively) for readying the body for action and slowing the body for deep rest and rejuvenation. Our body's reaction to external stimulation or perceived threat is to activate the sympathetic nervous system; in extreme situations this activation trips the "fight, flight, or freeze" response. Too much time spent in this state of hyperarousal causes the body to deteriorate. When the sympathetic nervous system is "on" for too long the endocrine glands become slow in their functioning, the immune system is weakened, and processes of physical recovery are impaired. The result can be sore muscles, excessive fatigue, or chronic minor disruptions of the body's metabolic processes that become cumulatively harmful. Individuals who are continually in a state of arousal deplete their body's reserves and become susceptible to a host of diseases as well as to heart dysfunction. We reestablish balance in the nervous system through diaphragmatic breathing, allowing the parasympathetic system to dominate for a time and to lead the body to rest, repair, and rejuvenate.

Diaphragmatic breathing has an immediate effect on mood and the level of calm a person experiences. Shallow chest breathing causes an excess of carbon dioxide in the bloodstream, which directly affects the acidity level of the blood. This imbalance of gases in the bloodstream can leave a person feeling tired, anxious, harried, and stressed. Chest breathing also causes an accumulation of muscle tension, particularly in the neck, upper back, shoulders, and between the shoulder blades. The jaw and facial muscles begin to show evidence of increased muscle tension. Often headaches and fatigue will present as accompanying symptoms.

When productive breathing patterns are in place the brain cells receive optimal supplies of oxygen, and this causes a person to feel vital, energetic, and serene. By breathing deeply we elicit the circulation of "feel-good hormones" throughout the brain and body and decrease muscle tension. How is this? Western scientists explain that the deep breathing undertaken during yoga practice stimulates the parasympathetic nervous system, which in turn decreases the production of stress chemicals, such as epinephrine, norepinephrine, and cortisol, and increases output of the "feel-good chemicals"—endorphins and serotonin.

Learning to breathe properly can change your life. Two of my students are prime examples of this.

Jennifer was a manager in a corporation being rocked by downsizing. After returning from vacation she found 200 e-mails in her inbox. That first week back from vacation Jennifer experienced tension headaches every day. New to the Yoga on the Ball classes, she decided she would try the diaphragmatic breathing she was learning in class. Jennifer would consciously "set her breath" the minute she sat down at her chair in the morning, and she would check her breath every time she answered the phone. From the very first day she employed what she called her "new breathing system" she developed no headaches. She now reports that she is a more serene, happier version of herself.

Vicky was a senior manager in the same corporation. Her job required her to fly often; every time she would climb into the company's helicopter she would become sick to her stomach. Vicky, too, decided to put to the test the new breathing she had learned in class. The next time she was required to travel via the company helicopter she practiced the long, slow yoga breathing pattern she was becoming familiar with in the Yoga on the Ball class. To her amazement the nausea never returned.

The athletes I work with accomplish far more with less effort when they figure out how to organize their breathing so that they breathe into both chest and belly during competition. I have found that the most effective way to teach athletes how to use the breath as a helpful performance tool is to first have them practice at rest. When they understand the concept of diaphragmatic breathing we then work on integrating it into their sport.

Correct breathing is as important to the person rehabilitating after an injury as it is to the athlete. Mary Massery, the world-famous physiotherapist who helped Christopher Reeve rehabilitate after his horseback riding accident, has designed an entire workshop about the healing effects of diaphragmatic breathing in relationship to rehabilitating injuries. Actively using the diaphragm in breathing provides the necessary precondition for taking the breath to the farthest reaches of the body, ensuring that the site of an injury is well nourished with oxygen and helping to keep the other systems working optimally, which promotes healing.

In following up with participants after a seminar the most frequent comment I hear is that yoga breathing has changed their lives. With increased awareness of their breathing patterns these students have learned how to monitor and modulate their breath throughout the day, leading to (among other things) fewer headaches, greater comfort through the neck and shoulders, an increased sense of calm and poise, less fatigue, and an ability to think clearly and creatively for longer periods of time. If any of these benefits sound appealing to you, most likely you could benefit from learning how to breathe differently. If you desire to experience more than one of these outcomes and you suffer from asthma, mood fluctuations, chronic pain, or other chronic conditions, the practice of diaphragmatic breathing could significantly influence the quality of your life.

When I encourage students to understand the huge benefits of changing the breath pattern from chest breathing to diaphragmatic, full-belly breathing, I often see a light of recognition go on in their eyes. People usually start out with a mild curiosity about yoga breathing techniques. After hearing about the wonderful benefits of diaphragmatic breathing and how vitalized it can make you feel, many students are thirsting to try it. Because of the demands placed on us by our fast-paced lives we crave solutions for managing our stress and developing optimal health that can be easily integrated into our lifestyles. The sumptuous cocktail of diaphragmatic breathing can be that much-needed tonic.

## Breath and Movement—The Dynamic Flow

Correct breathing is essential for the health of the mind and the body, and it becomes even more crucial when the body is under physical exertion. Diaphragmatic breathing helps to improve muscle endurance and keep the lungs and the heart moving smoothly and efficiently. Learning diaphragmatic breathing and pairing it with movement patterns can be challenging. In beginning a Yoga on the Ball practice many students breathe backward—puffing out the upper chest and drawing the belly in on the inhale—or find it difficult to pair the breath with the movement patterns. Many students have shared with me that their biggest challenge is continuing to breathe rhythmically when holding a challenging posture. Other students find it difficult to completely empty the lungs, which is essential for taking a full, deep gulp of fresh oxygen with the next breath.

What follows is a series of exercises designed to introduce you to diaphragmatic breathing. You will be encouraged to focus your attention on different areas of the trunk in these exercises, to encourage the movement of the diaphragm and to help the breath find its way into the deepest parts of the lungs. When learning these breathing practices have patience with yourself. Practice with curiosity, not judgment. An important part of practicing yoga is learning to honor yourself. Let this workout meet you where you are. Pay attention to your body by listening to the signals it communicates to you. The breath can serve as a barometer about how well you are tolerating the exercise. If you find your breathing becoming labored or find that you cannot perform a posture without holding your breath then the posture needs to be modified so that it is less demanding on your body. Or you need to take up yoga's resting pose—the Child pose—or another resting pose until you regain your steam.

Working with the breath and pairing it with movement creates fluidity in our motion and a sense of "being one" with the ball. In practicing yoga asanas the breath creates the bridge between one movement and the next. We begin our Yoga on the Ball practice by becoming aware of the breath. We then focus on consciously slowing it down, lengthening the inhalation and exhalation. Finally, we initiate pairing the breath with the movement patterns. Typically we expand a pose, or open up the body, on an inhale, and fold the body and bring the limbs closer to the trunk on the exhale.

As you become familiar with diaphragmatic breathing and what it has to offer you may find yourself actually looking forward to commencing your Yoga on the Ball practice with breathwork. I recommend that you begin every Yoga on the Ball workout with a breathing session. As you become familiar with the breathing practices, experiment with them. After you have exhaled all of your breath, focus on the peace and stillness that is present before the next breath comes in. Count silently while you inhale and exhale to slow and lengthen your breath, and observe how the natural length of the breath changes from day to day. Take note of how you feel when you consciously work with your breath.

The first breathing exercise in the practice section of this chapter focuses on observing the properties of the breath. Once we are able to identify our breathing patterns we can then learn to adjust them so that we can benefit from full-belly, diaphragmatic breathing. When we are under pressure we tend to breathe shallowly and quickly; parts of the inhalation phase and exhalation phase become choppy, uneven, ragged. You may find places in your inhalation/exhalation cycle where your breath catches, places where you stop breathing for a split second or more. You may observe that you sigh frequently when you have a tight deadline for a project at work. You might even notice that you have several different kinds of sighs, all relating to very different emotions. Lately I have noticed that I sigh one way when I am feeling pressured, yet I sigh a completely different way when I am feeling sad or disappointed. What does sighing have to do with breathing? Sighs are a breathing pattern—a stress-related breathing pattern, but a pattern nonetheless. Our

21

breathing patterns can give us useful information about our emotions and our soul stirrings.

Once we become experienced at detecting our gross breathing patterns we can begin to work toward making even subtle changes in our inhalations and exhalations. On the other hand, if we do not notice that we are breathing quickly in a choppy, less-than-optimal pattern and we do not make conscious attempts to slow, lengthen, and smooth out the breath, it then becomes habit to breathe incorrectly, even when we are not under stress. Most people are amazed at what they discover when they begin to monitor their breathing patterns.

Once we know what our breathing patterns are we can direct our efforts toward improving them when and where necessary, like Vicky breathing calmly before she flies on her business trips or like parents who slow down their breath to gather themselves before correcting their child's behavior. The goal of breathwork is to get rid of all the "raggedy edges" in the breath cycle, making the breaths smooth and calm and encouraging an adequate length of time to accommodate a relaxed inhalation and exhalation phase.

When we breathe smoothly and calmly our bodies spend more time operating out of the restful parasympathetic system. We all have those times when we struggle with a project, an assignment, or even a challenging family situation or business meeting, and of course the more we struggle the faster our breathing and pulse rate become, causing the sympathetic nervous system's "fight or flight" reaction to intensify. Operating from this fight or flight mode makes us less effective.

Actively practicing diaphragmatic breathing can take us to a calmer state of mind. A teaching tenet from India states that when the breath wanders the mind is unsteady, but when the breath is still so is the mind. When we are calm and relaxed we are more creative and clear thinking and are more likely to experience flashes of inspiration or vision. In this less aroused physiological state we are more likely to generate a wide variety of solutions to problems and are more likely to choose the most adaptive positive response available to us in any given moment. From the serene state in which we ride the soothing wave of the ebb and flow of the diaphragmatic breath we find the Divine, the mystery of spirit and soul.

Most spiritual teachers recommend that focusing on the breath is the first step toward accessing spirit (our own and the divine spirit) so that we can move toward *sadhana*, communion with God, or the kindhearted Great Mystery. Some religions encourage people to feel the spirit of this Great Mystery entering the body as the pace of the breath slows and the body relaxes. The breath is a scriptural symbol of the presence of God's spirit. Many people report to me that it is when they are enraptured with the movement of the breath flowing in and out of the body that they feel a connection with a divine presence, or with their highest self. Others tell me that focusing on the movement of the breath in the body becomes a numinous experience at times, and they receive answers to prayers or spiritual questions they've been asking. Still others have shared that when they are moving into a spiritual moment while working with the breath images of eagles or mountains or some other empowering symbol flash into their mind's eye. This kind of clarity and insight is common in the practice of yoga.

One of my favorite exercises is to sit on the ball in front of a window so that I can drink in the magnificence of the vast sky above. I use a soft gaze and focus on slowing my breath. For me this is a first step toward opening my heart to allow the spirit of the Divine to be ushered in. I often start my day this way, to bless the day ahead of me so that all of my projects and my relations will reflect the Divine's desires for my behavior and to pave the way for inspiration. Sometimes I end the day the same way, sitting on my ball looking up at the stars, slowing my breathing, and thanking God for all the blessings of the day.

## Yoga Breath and Ballwork

Yoga on the Ball practice can begin with the following breathing exercises. They help orient the mind to the present moment and prepare the body for the workout ahead. They can also be valuable tools to have in your stress management kit. If you have had a rough day and are feeling particularly anxious you may want to practice these exercises alone as a way to rejuvenate. If you have a ball at work you may want to practice this exercise during the day, whenever you feel tired or stressed. Because it promotes clear thinking, deep, diaphragmatic breathing is also a useful exercise for helping prepare the mind for an important meeting.

In working with these exercises you will want to pay close attention to any sensations you experience as your breath moves in and out of your body. You might consider starting a journaling process to track your progress and experiences with respect to breath training. You may want to record notes about the properties of your breath—short descriptions such as "choppy," "smooth," "sighing," "wheezing," "blocked," "jerky," "fluid"—as well as notes on how many seconds your inhalation and exhalation phase lasted. These notes can help you establish a baseline for use in tracking your progress with your breath training and can also help guide you in noticing how your breath relates to your emotions. The breath can give us good cues about how we might adjust our lifestyle to be more healthful and less stressful.

## Breath Check

This Breath Check exercise will help you become acquainted with the properties of the breath. The light pressure of the ball on the trunk helps you to focus on the area where the breath most noticeably moves through the body. Start there, focusing on how your body responds as breath moves in and out. Observing the flow of the breath can help you get a measure of your physiological and psychological state of being. If you are anxious and worried you may find that you breathe short, shallow breaths punctuated by sighs. You might observe places in your breathing cycle where your breath catches or you feel like gasping. Conversely, when you are relaxed and optimistic the breath tends to flow more smoothly and easily, and the length of the inhale approximates that of the exhale. This is the place in your practice where you may want to begin recording your experiences in a journal as you tune your attentions to your breath.

**Purpose** To help you focus closely on the properties of your breath.

**Watchpoints** • Lie comfortably on the floor. Be sure to maintain the natural curve of your low back. • Focus your mind on your breathing patterns.

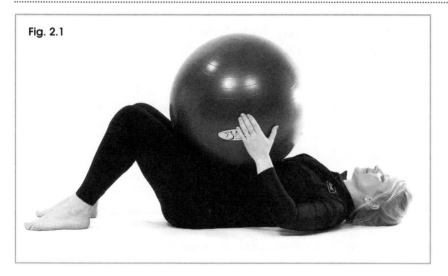

**Fig. 2.1**

*starting position*

Lie on your back. Place the ball on your belly and secure it with your hands (fig. 2.1).

*movement*

**1.** For your first five breath cycles, focus your attention on the movement of your belly as the breath moves in and out of your body.

**2.** For the next five breath cycles notice how the ball moves as you inhale and exhale.

**3.** Now ask yourself the following questions:

Are my inhalations long and slow or short and choppy? Are there any places where my breath catches? Did I sigh while breathing, or do I feel like sighing now? Does the length of my exhale match the length of my inhale?

Are there times during my breathing cycle when my breath is ragged and uneven? You may want to make notes about the properties of your breath in a journal before moving on to the next exercise.

## *Diaphragmatic Breathing*

This next exercise will illustrate the process of diaphragmatic breathing. The gentle weight of the ball helps to promote awareness of how the low belly and the diaphragm muscle are moving. The ball also assists in encouraging muscle "memory" with respect to the diaphragm and its best use in breathing. At the end of this exploration notice any differences in how you feel compared with how you felt before you started. You may want to experiment with finding and focusing in the pause between the breaths, where there is profound stillness, quiet, and peace.

**Purpose** To experience diaphragmatic breathing and the movement of the abdomen in relationship to the diaphragm.

**Watchpoint** • Keep the back in a neutral position, maintaining the natural curve in the low back.

........................................................................................................................................

*starting position*

Lie on your back with the soles of your feet flat on the floor. Place the ball on your low belly and support it there with your hands (fig. 2.2). (Rearrange your feet if necessary so that the ball can rest at the lowest point of your belly.)

*movement*

**1.** Inhale deeply through the nose. Take the breath all the way down to the lowest part of your abdomen and allow the belly to swell like a balloon. Notice the ball rising as you fill the low belly with breath.

**2.** Exhale slowly through the mouth as you draw the belly in toward the spine. Notice the ball lowering as you draw the belly in and release the breath.

**3.** Repeat for several breaths.

**4.** Now begin to elongate the breath, attempt-

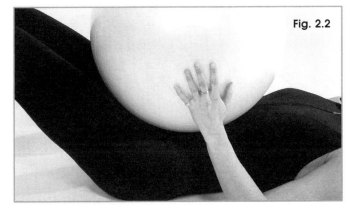

Fig. 2.2

ing to inhale and exhale to the count of ten. (When you become practiced at diaphragmatic breathing you will be able to both inhale and exhale through the nose while maintaining this deep belly breathing.) Stay here for as long as it's comfortable, usually 1 to 3 minutes. Savor any good feelings or pleasurable sensations you may be experiencing in your body.

# Modified Child Pose (Mudhasana)

This asana provides you with a rest pose that you can use whenever you feel you need to take a break during or after your workout. It stretches the erector spinae, the muscles that extend the entire length of the spine that often become tight and sore, riddled with tension. This is also an excellent exercise for relieving muscle tension in the back that can result from sitting for long periods of time at a desk or computer.

**Purpose** To provide a rest posture that you can assume between challenging postures or at the end of a workout. To stretch the erector spinae.

**Watchpoints** • Do not lock the elbows. • Discontinue this pose if you have trouble with your knees.

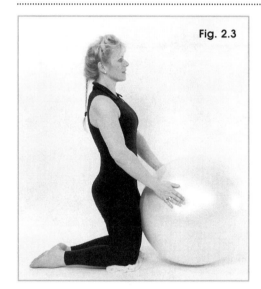

Fig. 2.3

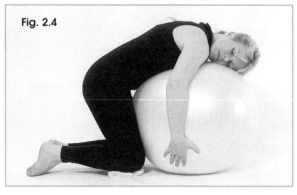

Fig. 2.4

*starting position*

Kneel on a mat or a folded towel with the ball in front of you, hands lightly resting on the top sides of the ball (fig. 2.3).

*movement*

**1.** Lean forward and drape your body over the ball (fig. 2.4). Surrender to allowing your spine and back to mould to the shape of the ball. Allow gravity to lengthen your spine; feel the traction-stretch through the upper and mid-back. Notice that the gentle stretch extends into the buttocks as well. Invite a release of tension throughout the length of the whole spine, including the base of the skull.
**2.** Practice diaphragmatic breathing, dropping the belly toward the floor on the inhale. Rest in this pose for as long as you need to.

# Prana Power

The next exercises set the foundation for helping pair the breath with movement. This one especially helps me to awaken the connection between my breath and the movement of my body. Typically in yoga we "open" the body, stretching the limbs away from the core, as we inhale, and we bring the limbs closer to the body on the exhale. In this exercise you will want to focus on the sensation of the body opening up through the chest and shoulders as you lift the ball overhead.

**Purpose** To train the body and brain to pair breath with movement. To demonstrate how the body "opens up" on the inhale and "closes" on the exhale.

**Watchpoints** • Do not arch the back off the floor. • Keep the elbows slightly bent.

*starting position*

Lie on your back with your knees bent, the soles of your feet on the floor. Set the ball on your belly and place your hands on either side of the ball.

*movement*

**1.** Inhale as you raise the ball up over your head and place it on the floor behind you (fig. 2.5). Be careful not to arch your back as you raise your arms. Remember to feel for the swell of the belly on the inhale.
**2.** Exhale as you lower the ball to the belly, back to the starting position. Feel the belly flatten on the exhale (fig. 2.6).
**3.** Repeat for four breath cycles.

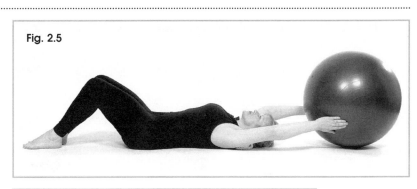

Fig. 2.5

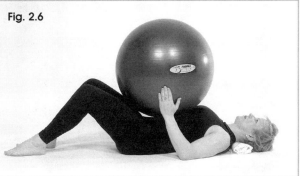

Fig. 2.6

## Prayer Breath

This rhythmical pairing of breath with movement helps to prepare you for the more intense yoga postures ahead. Anytime you place your hands in prayer position in yoga practice it is a sign of respect and reverence. In group practice it is customary to make a slight bow to the other practitioners while holding the hands in prayer position. Often this is accompanied by saying "Namaste," which means "the light in me (or 'the God in me') bows to the light in you."

In Yoga on the Ball, prayer position is a moving asana. Notice how the body opens up and stretches as the arms move overhead. As the arms come back in toward the body, focus on the place where the feet touch the ground to help you anchor and center yourself for the work ahead.

**Purpose** This breathing pattern helps to center and ground you before commencing your asana practice.

**Watchpoints** • Elongate the spine. • Position your body weight in the center of your ball so you do not lose your balance when you lift your arms overhead.

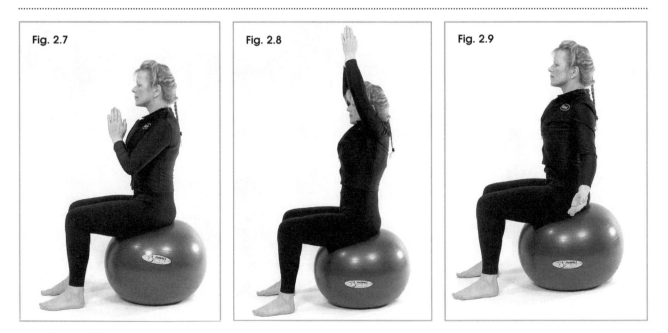

Fig. 2.7    Fig. 2.8    Fig. 2.9

*starting position*

Sit tall on the ball, feet shoulder-distance apart, toes point forward, ankle joints aligned below the knees. Bring your hands together at your chest in prayer position (fig. 2.7).

*movement*

**1.** Maintaining your hands in prayer position, inhale as you reach your arms overhead (fig. 2.8).

**2.** Exhale as you release the arms to your sides (fig. 2.9) and back to the chest in prayer position.
**3.** Repeat this moving asana three to five times.

Review this section and practice the breathing exercises until you become familiar with diaphragmatic breathing and pairing breath with movement. As you move further into the book revisit this chapter until you are able to fully integrate the breath with the Yoga on the Ball exercises.

Begin to institute periodic "breath checks" throughout your day. Bring your awareness to the breath. Are you performing shallow chest breathing? Or are you making full use of your diaphragm by breathing full, deep exhalations? Ask yourself: "Is my breathing pattern choppy and shallow or deep and rhythmic? Am I gasping or sighing? Is there any place during the respiration cycle where my breath feels ragged and uneven? Are my inhalations and exhalations long and deep? Does my inhalation match my exhalation?" Consciously practice deep diaphragmatic breathing whenever you think of it during your day, especially when you are in situations that make you anxious—driving in heavy traffic, preparing for a meeting, waiting in a long line, meeting with your boss.

Place your ball in your living space or use it as your chair at work so that when you need to take some time out to rest or regroup your ball is easily accessible. Rest on the ball as you practice conscious breathing. Roll on the ball, letting it massage your muscles. Let the ball help you find your body's tight spots. Send the breath into those areas that are sore. Rest, breathe, regenerate—feel the soft cushioned support underneath you as you drink in the tantalizing elixir of full and deep oxygenated breaths.

# 3

# Finding Postural Ease with Yoga Ball Asanas

In the previous chapter we discussed the importance of diaphragm movement in breathing and how to encourage full-belly, diaphragmatic breathing patterns. In order to practice healthy breathing patterns the spine and the skeleton must be in easy, effortless alignment. In this chapter we'll learn what constitutes good alignment. You will be hearing about neutral spine, neutral pelvis, and neutrality in the joints—all hallmarks of ideal posture.

Prana, the body's vital energy, must be able to circulate freely in order for a person to enjoy optimum health. Prana moves easily through a body that is erect in stature, one in which the chest is open and the shoulders and chin are gently retracted. A misaligned skeleton can be an obstacle to the strong flow of this life energy. When we sit, stand, or move in ways that don't maintain the integrity of the body's optimal alignment we block the flow of prana through the body.

In this chapter you will learn a set of yogic tools that will help you gain a clear understanding of what optimal alignment entails and how to cultivate healthy postural habits.

## Ellie's Story

Ellie is a woman not unusual in today's world. An advertising executive, Ellie waited until she was well established in her career before beginning a family.

She took full advantage of the maternity leave that allowed her to enjoy her new baby and helped her slowly get used to her new role and all of the responsibilities associated with motherhood.

Ellie scheduled an appointment with me shortly after she returned to work. She felt she was developing a nice rhythm in her life, one that allowed her to manage both her career and motherhood. Ellie was now ready to begin working toward developing a fitness routine that would fit easily into the life she was creating for herself.

Ellie had been in superb shape prior to her pregnancy. Now she wanted not only to regain her former fitness level but also wanted me to furnish some suggestions that might help alleviate the pain that had begun creeping into her neck, shoulders, and upper back. She reported that since going back to work the right side of her body ached with some consistency. She was not only experiencing pain during the workday but also while walking to work and during the middle of the night, in the hours she was attempting to get a new mom's much-needed rest.

Before designing Ellie's fitness routine we examined the ways in which she carried out the activities of her daily life. Ellie's muscles had suffered somewhat from the hiatus she had taken from her workouts—she simply did not have the muscle strength and balance she had prior to baby Matthew coming onto the scene. In carrying a baby, nursing, and pushing a stroller Ellie was using muscles in ways that were further creating imbalance in her upper body. As well, Ellie frequently sat for long hours in front of a computer or driving to business meetings. These work activities were contributing to her muscle imbalance.

The very first task Ellie and I undertook was retraining her muscles so she could learn to sit in and maintain ideal alignment while at work, while driving to business meetings, while nursing Matthew, or even while watching television. Ellie was to keep an exercise ball both at home and at work so that she could perform exercises that would help to train her postural muscles and improve muscle balance. I encouraged Ellie to sit on the exercise ball as often as she could, including when she was working at her desk or watching television at day's end. The very act of sitting on the ball activates the deep stabilizing muscles along the spine, muscles that help to support the body in ideal alignment.

The ball provided Ellie with a means for addressing her need for balance in her lower leg muscles as well. Ellie found that her calf muscles and her Achilles' tendons were frequently sore and tender—Ellie's Achilles' tendons had been dramatically shortened as a result of wearing high-heeled shoes. We helped Ellie define ways to lengthen the tendon by using the exercise ball, positioning herself over the ball in Plank pose and pressing her heels to the floor.

As she realized the impact that her shoe choices had on her calf muscles, Ellie chose to begin wearing supportive running shoes for her long jaunt to the office and whenever possible during the day. The high heels she began carrying in a backpack, which she substituted for her briefcase. That was the second "a ha" for Ellie as she began exploring the physical ramifications of her daily life. Ellie was in the habit of walking downtown to her office every day, always accompanied by an overstuffed briefcase carried in her right hand. By the time she got to the office the top of her right shoulder was filled with searing pain. By the end of the day Ellie's neck, both shoulders, and her upper back were fatigued and in spasm.

In addition to shortening her Achilles' tendon the high heels were pulling Ellie's spine out of alignment and creating muscular imbalance in the shoulders. The right shoulder, which carried her overstuffed briefcase, was much stronger than the left; the only way Ellie could convey the heavy case was by hanging on to the handle with her right hand and wearing the long carrying strap over her right shoulder. The backpack that Ellie switched to would serve a few purposes. First, it would help maintain ideal alignment in the spine by gently pulling her shoulders back rather than hunched and rolling forward; the backpack would also help to keep her shoulders level. Second, the strap of a briefcase would no longer be tearing into Ellie's shoulder and causing local muscle irritation and neck and upper back pain. The backpack we chose for Ellie had wheels so she could pull it along when navigating through a building or an airport, as long as she alternated arms frequently. Otherwise neck and shoulder problems would continue to prevail due to overuse on one side of the body.

If Ellie had been able to maintain an uninterrupted schedule in her fitness routine she could have counteracted and prevented the effects of the new demands placed on her upper body by making simple adjustments to her workout regime. As it was it took some time before we could reestablish the appropriate muscle balance in Ellie's body. We began that process by designing Ellie's fitness routine so that she avoided any exercises that would strengthen the chest and the front of the shoulders, as these muscles were already tight due to her daily activities. We concentrated instead on strengthening the back and the posterior shoulders.

With the use of the exercise ball Ellie began to establish balance in the spinal muscles by integrating back-extension exercises, such as the Cobra and other yoga postures, into her routine. Strengthening the posterior shoulder muscles was accomplished by lifting and lowering the hips while in a reverse yoga Plank position. We strengthened Ellie's midback with repetitions of scapula retraction while in Half Plank. The Fish pose, with arm variations, was perfect for opening the body and developing flexibility in the chest and front shoulder muscles.

Once we had some exercises in place that addressed Ellie's muscle imbalances we were able to fine-tune her fitness routine. Proceeding to her fitness regimen without addressing her postural needs would have left Ellie prone to further injury.

## The Importance of Balanced Posture

Erect posture makes a person look taller and more physically "together"; it also helps prevent unnecessary wear and tear on the body. Posture can even display our moods. Collapsed posture can signal a depressed, discouraged state of mind, whereas an easy vertical posture suggests confidence and present-moment attention. When we sit or stand present and aligned we breathe better, because the lungs have more room to expand within the rib cage. Breathing oxygenates the brain, lowering anxiety and creating a positive state of mind. Often simply shifting the spine in order to stand or sit taller can make us feel empowered and optimistic.

Prana moves through the body most freely when the bones and joints are in proper alignment. With prana pulsing through the body's energy centers, what yogis call the *chakras*, every cell is healthier and more vibrant. The mind is sharper and more focused, and the nervous system functions more effectively. We are more in touch with our intuition and the spiritual realm. Yogic theory tells us that in this state we become connected with a divine intelligence—something beyond our own personal power, a nexus in which synchronicity and serendipity prevail. Yogis believe that in this state we are more able to actualize and move toward our highest potential and personal destiny in this life.

It is not only the five-thousand-year-old disciplines of yoga and martial arts that dictate the value of optimal posture. More recent bodywork practices, such as rolfing and the neuromuscular practices developed by Moshe Feldenkrais, F. M. Alexander, and Joseph Pilates, also sing the praises of good body posture.

Postural deviations caused by abnormalities in the bones cannot be improved by exercise and are permanent. However, when poor posture is a result of muscle imbalance and lack of postural awareness we can correct the deviation with education and appropriate exercise.

33

## Ideal Alignment

The adult vertebral column consists of thirty-three vertebrae divided into five groups. The upper seven are the cervical vertebrae; the twelve that follow are called the thoracic vertebrae; the next five are the lumbar vertebrae. Below the lumbar spine is the sacrum, consisting of five vertebrae that are fused together. The coccyx, also known as the tailbone, is comprised of four vertebrae stacked one on top of the other at the very base of the spine.

When properly aligned the spine of an adult has three natural, gentle curves. In this position, called "neutral spine," the pressure on the spongy discs between each vertebrae is equalized. The discs are not squeezed or displaced to the back or the front, such as happens when we slouch or when we hyperextend the spine. Whether sitting, standing, or lying down, it is beneficial to maintain the integrity of the spine by aligning the spinal column to reflect this natural curvature.

A neutral pelvis functions like a neutral spine in that it protects the spine from injury by preventing the discs from becoming compressed. To more effectively understand the concept of neutral pelvis visualize the pelvis as if it were a bucket of water. In the anterior-tilt (or front-tilt) position water would tip out of the front of the bucket. Similarly, in a posterior-tilt position water would tip out the back of the bucket. In neutral position the bucket would be level and therefore there would be no spillage.

When first learning the concept of neutral pelvis some students benefit from placing a ball on the belly and observing which way the ball rolls—this tells you if you are in a posterior tilt or an anterior tilt at the moment. The ball balances on the belly when the pelvis is aligned in neutral.

When I am teaching neutral position to the child athletes I train I ask them to lie on the floor and try to create a flat table with the pelvis, a table on which they could have a tea party. This type of cueing seems to create a clear visual picture of the concept I am trying to explain and is quite effective in bringing about proper positioning. You may want to use some sort of visual cueing for yourself. I like to visualize imaginary lines joining the hipbones with the pubic bone to create a flat triangular shape. This way I can sense whether I have created a level plane by the positioning of these bones.

It does not matter if you are standing, sitting, or lying down, once you train your brain to visualize the lines needed to achieve neutral pelvis and adjust your bones accordingly, you can create neutral pelvis.

Once you understand the concept of neutral pelvis you may find yourself doing your own postural "studies" on the street. One of the classic postural deviations I notice is when I am observing our young people. The next time you see kids hanging out together see if you can spot this too. It is typical to see teens wearing oversized jeans held up by the top crest of the hipbone. Those bony hips are usually drawn backward into a posterior pelvic tilt, which thrusts the pubic bone forward. This posture can have its rewards if your name is Elvis Presley or Tom Jones, but if you "live" in this posture you are doing yourself harm. With the hips constantly held in a posterior tilt the hamstrings shorten, which, in turn, brings about a flat-back posture. In this position the vertebrae of the spine are misaligned and the person is left vulnerable to injury.

Conversely, if you are one of those people who has an excessive anterior tilt your hipbones will be thrust forward and your tailbone will be pressed out behind you. This pelvic position increases the inward curve of the low back. When you observe people with this postural deviation you will notice that quite often it is associated with a protruding abdomen and buttocks, along

## The Neutral Pelvis and Spine

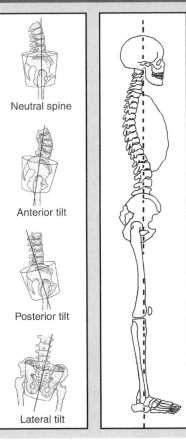

*t*he pelvis and spine are in neutral position when neither structure is rotated or tipped in any direction. Pelvic positioning is classified as anterior when the lumbar spine is hyperextended and the pubic bone is drawn back. When the pelvis is imagined as a bucket, in anterior tilt water would spill out of the front of the bucket. In posterior tilt the hip is hyperextended and the pubic bone presses forward. Water would spill out of the back of the bucket in this positioning of the pelvis. When the pelvis is laterally tilted the hips are horizontally uneven; in the bucket analogy water spills out the side.

In optimal alignment the pelvis is level side to side and anchored in a central position between the two extremes of

Neutral spine

Anterior tilt

Posterior tilt

Lateral tilt

posterior and anterior tilt. This positioning provides a balanced base for the alignment of the spinal column.

Observing a well-aligned spine and pelvis from a side view you could draw a plumb line that would pass through various structures of the body. Following gravity the plumb line would pass through the middle of the ear and then bisect the center of the shoulder, hip, and knee joints, culminating in a spot directly in front of the ankle joint. In this alignment all joints reflect a state of neutrality, with each side of the body being a mirror image of the other. The balanced dynamics of this skeletal alignment provides a structure from which the body can move most efficiently and protects the key joints of the spine and pelvis from injury.

with rounded shoulders and a forward head posture. This spinal alignment leads to compression of the discs on one side of the lumbar and cervical spine. This forces the discs to protrude from the other side of the vertebral spine. If this postural positioning is left unchecked these bulging discs can result in further problems. They can be "pinched off" during the simple flexion or extension moves of everyday activities, and this herniated disc material can then press into the nerves of the spinal cord, a condition that causes excruciating pain. When postural deviations bring about problems of this magnitude often surgery is the only recourse. People so afflicted often require a medication cocktail just to tolerate the pain, and they may find that there is no position in which the pain is completely absent.

Some people have pelvises that are not level. This most often is the result of standing with one hip jutted out to the side. You might notice in your conversations with people you know well and interact with a lot that they tend to favor jutting one hip out to the side. This presentation is known as a lateral pelvic tilt. I have often noticed in women who have young children that you can guess which hip they balance their babies on because that hip will be higher than the other. When this hip jutting becomes habitual in a person's stance the muscles on the side of the hip that juts out become overstretched and the muscles on the other side become shortened. This sort of imbalance in the hips can transfer downward to the knee and ankle musculature, affecting the person's gait and leaving her vulnerable to injury at the knee and ankle joints.

The next important concept of good spinal alignment that I want to draw your attention to is transverse abdominis activation. We first discussed the transverse abdominis in chapter 2 in its role as part of the body's core musculature. An active transverse abdominis muscle provides an enlivened corset of protection for the spine. We activate the transverse abdominis by drawing the belly button up and in toward the spine. (This action is best executed on the exhalation phase of your breathing cycle.) The simple action of drawing the navel toward the spine helps to align the spine and to maintain its position.

When you anchor the spine in optimal alignment you have a solid and sturdy base from which to generate power in your movements. Learning to properly use the musculature of your transverse abdominis helps you to center in the strong core of your body so that all your movements originate from this sturdy, dependable foundation. Your movement patterns become more controlled, precise, and deliberate. When a person attempts to initiate movement without activating the transverse abdominis it can be likened to beating a rug while standing on ice. If we were watching someone doing such a thing we would observe flailing, unorganized, imprecise movement resulting in weak and ineffectual contact with the rug.

It is imperative that the spine be anchored in place before any movement is undertaken. When the spine is not supported by an active transverse abdominis the vertebrae and discs can slip out of place from the momentum of the movement, resulting in injury to the low back. And learning to properly engage the transverse abdominis not only helps to safeguard the spine but the simple act of drawing belly to spine tones the abdominal musculature, helping to develop an aesthetically pleasing look to the abdominals. Observing a side profile of a person activating his transverse abdominis you will notice a streamlined trunk and a "cinched" appearance to the waist.

The action that engages the transverse abdominis muscle is known to yogis as *uddiyana bhanda. Julandhara bhanda* is engaged by retracting the chin. *Mula bhanda* is executed by contracting the perineum. In traditional yoga practice work with the bhandas is paired with pranayama (breathwork) for the purpose of directing prana in the body so as to convert it to spiritual energy. Generally, practicing the bhandas would not take place until the yoga student had purified himself with several months of asana practice. Also, some yogis encourage the engagement of the bhandas in meditation in order to help treat various medical conditions. Use of the bhandas in this manner is beyond the scope of this book, but if you wish to know more about this fascinating subject I suggest you consult *Meditation as Medicine* by Dharma Singh Khalsa, M.D. In Yoga on the Ball bhanda work is undertaken in the beginning of the practice in order to coax the body into effortless and supported alignment.

When you activate the transverse abdominis in Yoga on the Ball poses you feel more relaxed and yet more secure in each asana because you have the solid sense that you are anchored to a strong base of support. In that moment we can sense we are striking the delicate balance between yoga *sukha*, steadiness, and *sthira*, ease of effort. Once you are used to working from your strong center you will find that you are able to create longer, straighter yoga lines throughout the body when practicing the asanas. Your yoga pose becomes more organized from the tip of your toes to the top of your head.

When you commit to aligning your body to support correct posture you will find that your breathing also becomes steady and less effortful. Posture and breath are essential ingredients of the solid foundation on which you can begin to build your personal Yoga on the Ball practice.

## *Postural Setup: Ideal Alignment*

As a prelude to working with Yoga on the Ball asanas you will want to balance the spine by practicing the bhandas and then align the body from the toes to the top of the head. We begin with the feet because it is advisable to always start your yoga practice by grounding yourself and moving into present-moment awareness—many people are assisted in this by contemplating the place where their feet connect with Mother Earth. The Postural Setup will take you step-by-step through the process of balancing the spine. You will want to work with the bhandas and scapular stabilization until the microadjustments they provide become second nature.

**Purpose** To arrange the spine in optimal alignment and center your weight evenly on the ball. To practice transverse abdominis activation for protecting the low back and for generating power.

**Watchpoints** • Keep tall through the spine. • Be careful not to suck the belly in by holding your breath.

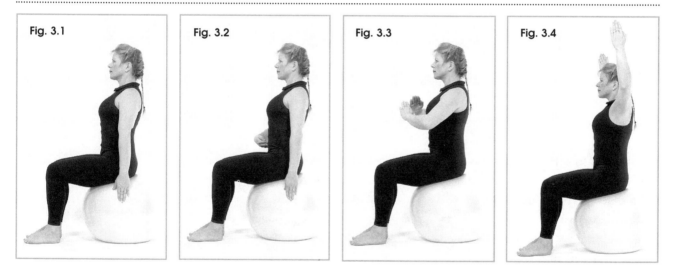

Fig. 3.1    Fig. 3.2    Fig. 3.3    Fig. 3.4

*starting position*

**1.** Begin by sitting tall on your ball, feet shoulder-width apart. The toes point forward, ankle joints aligned below the knees. Focus into the place where your feet connect with the earth (fig. 3.1).
**2.** Moving your awareness up your body, align your hips with your knees.
**3.** Place one hand on your low belly and draw your spine toward your navel, activating the band of muscle that wraps around your waist and protects your low back (fig. 3.2).

*movement 1: chest opener*

**1.** Cross the wrists at the heart chakra, the center of the chest (fig. 3.3). Inhale and draw the arms overhead (fig. 3.4).

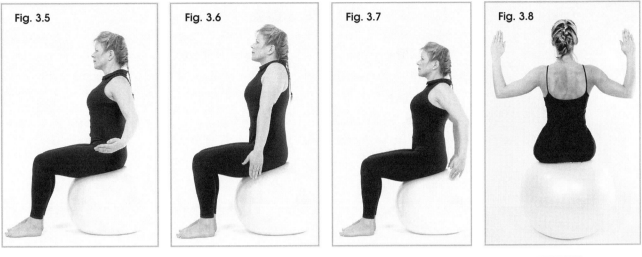

Fig. 3.5    Fig. 3.6    Fig. 3.7    Fig. 3.8

**2.** Exhale as you release the arms to your side (fig. 3.5). Make sure that your chest is lifted and your shoulders are not rounded.

**3.** Inhale as you lift the shoulders up (fig. 3.6), then roll your shoulders back as you exhale with a long "ahhhhhhhhhhh-hhh!" (fig. 3.7).

**4.** Repeat if you wish.

## movement 2: scapular stabilization

Use the muscles that reside between your shoulder blades to gently draw the shoulder blades together, stabilizing the scapula (fig. 3.8).

## movement 3: chin retraction (julandhara bhanda)

**1.** Now roll your shoulders back, place your fingers on your chin, and gently guide your head back and up (fig. 3.9). Yogis refer to this movement as juland-hara bhanda.

**2.** Find your yoga *dristi,* a point of focus, on the wall in front of you. Focus your gaze on that landmark. Using your vision in this way will further enhance your posture by keeping your chin properly aligned, neither dropping to the floor nor pointing toward the ceiling (fig. 3.10).

**3.** Notice where your head is situated

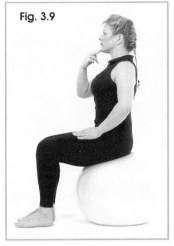

Fig. 3.9

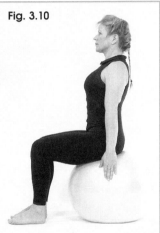

Fig. 3.10

relative to the top of the spine. Is your head bent forward? Is it tipped to one side or the other? Can you sense any imbalances here?

**4.** Now attempt to lengthen your neck and grow even taller. Feel your entire spine lengthen. Imagine that you are pressing the top of your head toward the ceiling so that the crown of your head and the ceiling will meet.

**5.** Take three diaphragmatic breaths, allowing your brain and nervous system to slowly integrate this postural pattern into its muscle memory.

## Tummy Compressions

The exercises below also provide you with several opportunities to more fully explore the activation of the transverse abdominis muscle. These transverse abdominis exercises provide ways to awaken what is for many a "sleepy" muscle. The exercises help you to find this important muscle and then work it.

**Purpose** To create muscle memory for activating the transverse abdominis muscle. To strengthen the transverse abdominis.

**Watchpoint** • Maintain the natural curve in the low back.

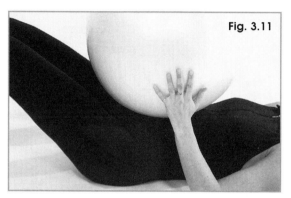

Fig. 3.11

*starting position*

1. Lie on your back with your knees bent and feet on the floor hip-distance apart. Lengthen the neck and ensure that the chin points toward the ceiling.

2. Place the ball on your low belly, supporting it with both hands (fig. 3.11).

*movement*

1. Inhale through the nose to fill the belly with air. Notice that the ball rises.
2. Exhale and draw the belly toward the spine. Notice that the ball sinks on the exhale.
3. As you breathe rhythmically, maintain a moderate contraction of the transverse abdominis (uddiyana bhanda) for approximately 6 seconds.
4. Inhale and gently release the contraction.
5. Repeat six to eight times.

## Half Plank with Uddiyana Bhanda

Half Plank with Uddiyana Bhanda helps to create awareness of and build strength in the transverse abdominis. This exercise builds on the Tummy Compressions, however it is slightly more challenging because the abdominals are working against gravity (which they were not doing in Tummy Compressions). Through this posture we learn that activating the transverse abdominis requires not only sinking the navel toward the spine but is about gently drawing the muscles in and up. Adding movement causes the muscles to work harder to stabilize the body.

**Purpose** To create awareness of and build strength in the transverse abdominis.

**Watchpoints** • Maintain a neutral spine throughout the posture. • Do not let the head droop.

### starting position

Drape the body over the ball in Half Plank position. Hands are palms down on either side of the ball directly beneath the shoulder joint; knees are beneath the hips. Be sure that your weight is distributed evenly on all four limbs. Maintain proper alignment of the head on the spine. Your gaze is at the floor.

### movement 1

**1.** Inhale and feel your belly press into the ball.
**2.** On the exhale activate the transverse abdominis (uddiyana bhanda) by drawing the navel upward and inward toward the spine, attempting to slightly lift the belly off the ball without moving the body.
**3.** Maintain this moderate contraction for 6 to 8 seconds as you breathe rhythmically.
**4.** Repeat six to eight times.

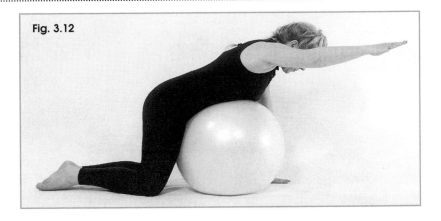

Fig. 3.12

### movement 2: add upper limbs

**1.** Inhale and feel the belly pressing into the ball.
**2.** On an exhale engage the transverse abdominis (uddiyana bhanda), drawing the belly upward and in toward the spine while you simultaneously lift one arm into Half Spinal Balance (fig. 3.12).

**3.** As you breathe rhythmically, maintain this moderate contraction for 6 to 8 seconds while holding the arm in the air.
**4.** Release the arm to the starting position.
**5.** Repeat on the other side.

# Abdominal Squeeze (Akunchan Prasarana)

This rhythmic abdominal exercise massages and improves circulation to the abdominal organs and dramatically changes the tone of the abdominal wall. The blood is squeezed out of the abdominal cavity on the exhale; on the inhale the abdominal cavity relaxes and a fresh supply of oxygen-rich blood is delivered to the organs. With this systematic pumping of the blood through the abdomen, the abdominal organs are revitalized; elimination, digestion, and absorption of nutrients is improved, and circulation increases.

When you first begin practicing this exercise you will want to generate a contraction that is approximately 30 percent of your maximum and then systematically increase the contraction to approximately 50 percent. Contracting at full power creates too much tension at the abdomen.

**Purpose** To strengthen the transverse abdominis muscle. To provide a gentle massage for the abdominal organs.

**Watchpoint** • Be sure to maintain the spine in a neutral position throughout this posture.

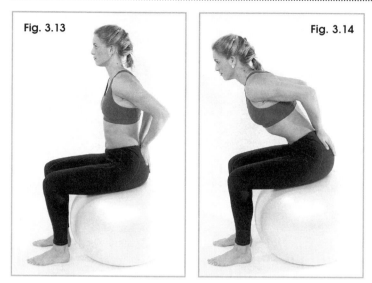

Fig. 3.13     Fig. 3.14

*starting position*

**1.** Sit on the ball with the feet placed a little more than hip-distance apart. Find neutral spine by using the Postural Setup.
**2.** Lean just slightly forward to place the palms of the hands on the sacroiliac joints on either side of the triangle-shaped sacrum at the base of the spine (fig. 3.13).

*movement*

**1.** Exhale and draw the belly button up and in toward the spine. Feel the transverse abdominis engage to about 30 percent of maximum contraction (fig. 3.14).
**2.** Release the belly to the start position on the inhale.
**3.** Repeat ten times.

# Meditative Yogi

This exercise will improve both your abdominal strength and your core stability. By balancing on the ball with one foot off the ground the abdominals are recruited in order to keep you from falling off the ball. This is a fun pose to practice and can make you smile trying.

**Purpose** To improve abdominal strength as well as balance.

**Watchpoints** • Sit tall in ideal alignment. • Breathe smoothly and calmly. • Strive to keep the hips level and still while you work through the movement.

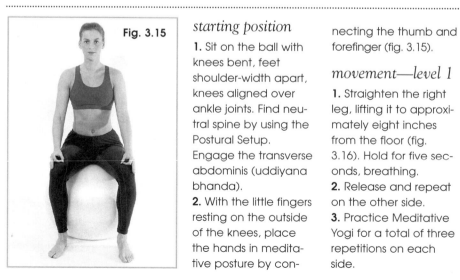

Fig. 3.15

*starting position*

**1.** Sit on the ball with knees bent, feet shoulder-width apart, knees aligned over ankle joints. Find neutral spine by using the Postural Setup. Engage the transverse abdominis (uddiyana bhanda).
**2.** With the little fingers resting on the outside of the knees, place the hands in meditative posture by con-necting the thumb and forefinger (fig. 3.15).

*movement—level 1*

**1.** Straighten the right leg, lifting it to approximately eight inches from the floor (fig. 3.16). Hold for five seconds, breathing.
**2.** Release and repeat on the other side.
**3.** Practice Meditative Yogi for a total of three repetitions on each side.

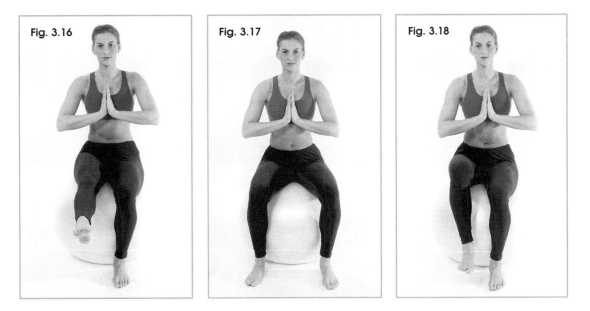

Fig. 3.16   Fig. 3.17   Fig. 3.18

## movement—level 2

**1.** Begin from the same starting position, using Postural Setup to find ideal alignment and engaging the transverse abdominis. Bring the hands in front of the breastbone and press the palms together in Prayer position (fig. 3.17).
**2.** Keeping the knee bent, lift the right foot approximately six inches off the floor (fig. 3.18). Hold for five seconds, breathing.

**3.** Place the right foot back on the floor. Before progressing to the left side make sure you are sitting in a balanced position and that the transverse abdominis is activated.
**4.** Repeat this movement on the left side of the body.
**5.** Place the left foot back on the floor. Check your posture.

You have now completed the Postural Setup and transverse abdominis activation and awareness exercises. I am amazed by how postural setting has become a part of my life—I now make adjustments to my posture without even thinking about it. My children laugh at me because I spontaneously align my spine and draw my navel toward my spine even before I bend to pick up something that has dropped to the floor—sometimes something as light as a piece of paper. I am guessing that you will find the same thing once you become familiar with these exercises—you may begin to notice that you align your spine and engage your abdominals before you turn to back in to the drive-way or before bending to take a dish out of the oven.

As you become familiar with the alignment and activation exercises, establish postural "awareness moments" in your daily routine—moments in which you trigger your attention toward checking the status of your abdominals. Maybe you'll want to make a habit of activating your abdominals when the phone rings. Or set your watch to remind you several times during the day to create slight tone in your low abdominals and ensure that you are not allowing the belly to protrude. These simple acts will help to tone and condition your transverse abdominis musculature so that you are able to steadily progress in your Yoga on the Ball program.

You can never go wrong by creating a slight bit of tone to ensure that the abdominals are not protruding. Individuals who are very deconditioned and have no awareness of activating the transverse abdominis run the risk of pulling the pelvis into an anterior tilt if they have an overly generous girth with very little tone. Once deconditioned individuals develop a higher base-line of tone in the transverse abdominis by holding a slight bit of activation at different times throughout the day, they will soon be able to engage the transverse abdominis for longer periods of time and with a far greater contraction.

As we have discussed throughout this chapter, enlivening the transverse abdominis leads to greater core stability, which protects the low back from injury and helps us move more efficiently and use our energy wisely. (And a pleasing side effect of an engaged transverse muscle is a more aesthetically pleasing, streamlined look to the abdominals.) Aligned and enlivened posture improves the way you sit, stand, and move as well as helps you to look better, feel better, and breathe better. Good posture will pay you great dividends for your entire life. You do yourself a great service by making postural checks a regular pattern in the movements of your life.

# 4

## That All-Important Warm-Up

Ask five different people what a warm-up is and you will likely get five completely different responses. Every time I visit the local fitness club to conduct a personal training I'm amazed at the variety of activities that people engage in as warm-up to exercise. For the most part what I see causes me concern.

The most common warm-up I see people performing at the gym is no warm-up at all. Countless times I have watched people arrive after work to join a friend for a squash or racquetball game, their sole warm-up being a set of one-sided shoulder rolls for the racquet arm or a couple of smashes of the ball against the wall. That's it for a game in which the heart can be pumping at more than 75 percent of its maximum rate in the first few minutes of play! It's enough to make my own heart race just thinking about it. I've witnessed people leave the court after being overwhelmed by dizziness, nausea, lightheadedness, and even chest pain—all potential signs of heart problems.

Sorrowfully, one member at the gym lost his life this way. It was early in the morning and a middle-aged man rushed onto the court so he could fit a game in before work. His squash partner and longtime buddy was chiding him about being late yet again. Both men were in superb shape and so simply began their game the moment John's feet hit the court floor.

They didn't even give their actions a second thought—a decision that proved tragic minutes later. You see, often in the first few minutes of an aerobic activity the heart will display unusual rhythms, especially if that heart resides in the chest of a middle-aged man. This phenomenon is even more accentuated if the activity is occurring first thing in the morning. When the circulatory system is warmed gradually and adequately the heart's rhythms will eventually even out, and the specter of impending doom is over.

On that cold winter morning death claimed John less than seven minutes after he arrived on the court. John started complaining of chest pain almost immediately after starting play that morning, but since both men boasted of their high level of conditioning neither one thought anything serious was occurring. John thought he was having gastrointestinal problems from eating his breakfast so quickly that morning. Phil thought John was horsing around and just kept playing and shooting verbal jabs at him. John dropped to the floor, writhing and twisting; even then Phil did not put it past his friend to keep the dramatics going. But then John's color changed to a horrible bluish gray. Within seconds John's eyes were lifeless.

Certainly this is a worst-case scenario, but even one tragedy such as this is one too many. It is a simple, workable commitment to your health to allow adequate time in your day for a thorough and appropriate warm-up, customized to suit the activity that you will be taking part in.

Why do we need to customize a warm-up? An appropriate warm-up gently engages the various body systems that will be in play during full-on activity. Different physical activities place different demands on different parts of the body; our warm-up must reflect the physical demands we'll be placing on our bodies during exercise. A warm-up prior to lifting weights should not be the same as a warm-up before pole vaulting. With weightlifting, stress is systematically placed on various muscles in the body, including the cardiac muscle. When pole vaulting the calf muscles take a noticeable beating due to the instantaneous concentric and eccentric contractions required of them. Gardening has different requirements than walking. In gardening a fair amount of strain can be placed on the hips, back, and wrists while cardiovascular output is mostly kept to a minimum. With walking the heart gets a moderate workout while stress to any one structure or muscle in the body is usually negligible (especially if your body is in good postural alignment!). It's important to analyze the demands of your activity and plan a warm-up that will help prevent the body from experiencing unnecessary stress or injury.

How do we determine what, in fact, is an appropriate warm-up? If you are preparing for a moderate to high-end aerobic activity it is advisable to exercise at a slower pace for eight to ten minutes, gradually approaching the heart-rate level you will ultimately work at. If you're in a cold environment or you are elderly, ten to fifteen minutes for a warm-up would be more appropriate.

A gradual warm-up prepares the muscles, heart, and lungs for the upcoming workload and increases the body's enzyme activity for the purpose of metabolizing fats and sugars more quickly so that energy can be made readily available. Also, lactic acid is less likely to pool in the joints when you warm up gradually. That means you will be less likely to experience the burning sensation in the limbs that often accompanies the preliminary stages of a workout. (Think of the times you warmed up too quickly—or not at all—and your arms and legs each seemed to weigh a ton when you were exercising. That is the effect of lactic acid buildup.) Finally, an efficient warm-up prepares your body to burn fat and helps to enhance your performance. All good things!

When the activity you're preparing for is a total-body form of exercise, such as yoga, it is most beneficial to warm up with a minimum of three to five minutes of continuous rhythmic activity. In this case our focus is on increasing the temperature in the muscles and in the tissues that connect muscle to bone and bone to bone. When muscles, tendons, and ligaments are warm they are more pliable and less vulnerable to injury. The heightened tissue temperature increases elasticity and flexibility. Warming these tissues also aids in shunting the blood from the spleen and stomach and to the working muscles, which require the extra oxygen and nutrients available from the increased blood flow.

Continuous, gentle, low-impact movement also increases the production of fluid in the synovial joints. This viscous fluid lubricates the joint, facilitating movement and decreasing the likelihood of the movement causing wear and tear at the joint.

I always find it useful to begin and end my Yoga on the Ball session with a few minutes of diaphragmatic breathing. I lie down on a rug or my yoga mat with a ball resting on top of my belly and simply focus on the sensation of the breath swelling my belly on the inhale and my navel dropping toward my spine on the exhale. I find it deeply relaxing to feel the gentle pressure of the ball on the belly as my breath swells and recedes. (Review chapter 2 for detailed guidance on breathing.) Diaphragmatic breathing and focusing on the sensations of the muscles as they warm helps bring the mind to the present moment, an important element of a yoga session.

To begin your Yoga on the Ball practice I suggest that you execute several rounds of diaphragmatic breathing in a reclining position. Then I recommend that you sit on your ball and continue to practice the relaxing cadence of the deep diaphragmatic breathing as you perform shoulder rolls to open the chest and expand the lungs. Next, take meticulous care with finding good skeletal alignment with the Postural Setup described in chapter 3; revisit the place where you identify your transverse abdominis musculature (uddiyana bhanda) and consciously engage these. I enjoy going through this sequence for the postural benefits as well as the relaxing physical benefits it provides.

My recommendation would now be for you to practice Prayer Breath, the fluid pairing of breath with movement that can help prepare you, physically and mentally, for the yoga postures ahead. Place your hands in prayer position at the heart chakra, inhale to raise your hands to the heavens, and exhale as you slowly lower your arms to your sides. (Prayer Breath is described fully in chapter 2). I find this sequence of breath and postural movements to be an effective way to ground and center myself as a first step in my yoga practice.

Most traditional forms of yoga begin with a flowing asana called Sun Salutation, or Surya Namaskar. Sun Salutation is a graceful sequence of linked yoga postures designed to create *tapas*, or heat, in the body and to prepare the mind and body for more extensive practice.

When practicing Sun Salutation as a warm-up we do not hold any of the poses for any more than the breath or two that it takes to fully execute each posture. With this constant rhythmic movement we are able to create the tapas necessary to help the body accommodate for the remainder of the practice.

In the full sequence of Sun Salutation, described below, pay close attention to the instructions given regarding breathing and body positioning. Practice each segment separately until you gradually become familiar with the entire sequence, and in no time you will be able to complete the entire Sun Salutation without constantly stopping and starting.

Once you become adept at practicing Sun Salutation you will find it an exhilarating process to move through. You can use this as an aerobic-conditioning exercise by performing several repetitions of Sun Salutation at a lively pace. If you wish to use your Yoga on the Ball program as a cardiovascular session you can do so by combining a lively paced Sun Salutation with other moving Yoga on the Ball asanas.

# Sun Salutation (Surya Namaskar)

Surya Namaskar is a yoga-specific warm-up designed to prepare both body and mind for more extensive asana practice. In the Yoga on the Ball program Surya Namaskar is executed completely on the ball. Honor your body by listening to the cues it provides you and set your practice pace accordingly. For instance, if you find that your breathing becomes labored or there are places where you are holding your breath during the Sun Salutation, you need to slow your pace. Similarly, if you feel tightness in some areas of your body as you move through the warm-up you will want to adjust your movements so that you are not pressing into the postures quite so intensely. Then set your workout pace according to your needs based on the sensations you feel as you move through the warm-up.

**Purpose** To heat the body, lubricate the joints, and prepare the muscles, connective tissue, heart, and lungs for more extensive strengthening and stretching asanas.

**Watchpoints** • As you move in and out of the various postures of Surya Namaskar, maintain impeccable form through the use of neutral posture and ideal alignment. • Some movements in Surya Namaskar can be difficult for people who are new to yoga or to ballwork, as they especially require strong abdominal engagement and good balance. Be patient with yourself and your ability to "flow" through Sun Salutation will develop. • The breath will help you link one posture to the next, making your movements more fluid.

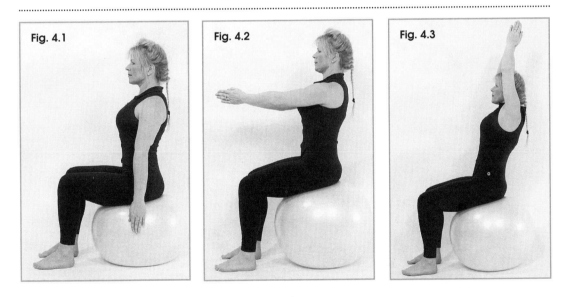

Fig. 4.1    Fig. 4.2    Fig. 4.3

*starting position*

**1.** Sit on the ball with your feet shoulder-width apart. Elongate and align the spine and retract your chin so that your head is sitting directly on top of your spine (fig. 4.1). Activate the muscles between your shoulder blades to draw your shoulders down and back.
**2.** Place your hands in prayer position at your breastbone.

*movement 1*

**1.** Inhale as you extend the arms in front of you, palms together (fig. 4.2).
**2.** On the exhale activate the transverse abdominis as you sweep the arms overhead to lean into a gentle backbend (fig. 4.3). Tip your head back slightly so that the head stays in line with the spine. The chin will lift a small amount.
**3.** Inhale in this gentle backbend, or Cobra asana.

49

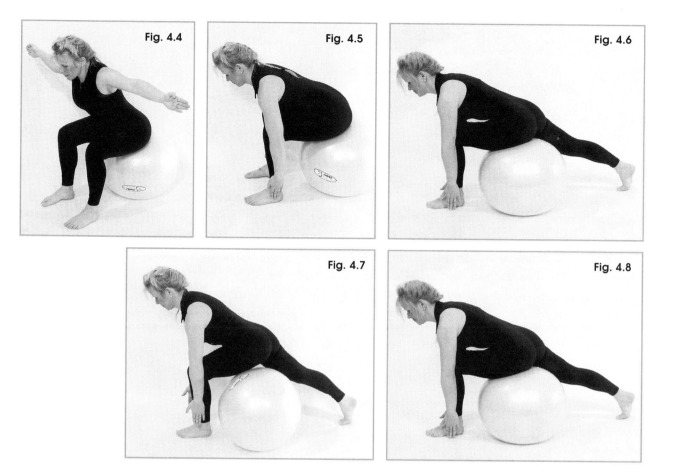

## movement 2

**1.** As you exhale, engage the transverse abdominis and fold at the hips to extend forward, arms out at the sides of the body (fig. 4.4). Stop at the point at which you begin to round the back.

**2.** Support the weight of your upper body in this position by placing your hands on your knees or beside your ankles (fig. 4.5). Make sure the spine is elongated and straight.

## movement 3

**1.** Breathe rhythmically as you shift the left foot so that it aligns with the center of your body.

**2.** Simultaneously extend the right leg back and fold forward at the hips to extend your hands toward the floor on either side of the left foot (fig. 4.6).

## movement 4

**1.** Inhale as you straighten the back (right) knee, lifting the hips off the ball (fig. 4.7). The lower part of the back thigh maintains only slight contact with the ball. Feel the stretch in the right groin and the front of the right thigh.

**2.** On an exhale engage the transverse abdominis as you bend the back knee slightly and deepen the sink of the front thigh, taking care not to bend that knee past 45 degrees (fig. 4.8).

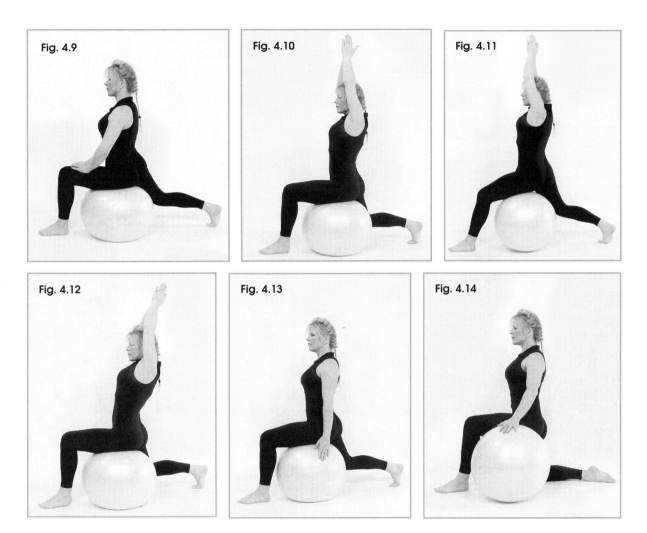

Fig. 4.9  Fig. 4.10  Fig. 4.11
Fig. 4.12  Fig. 4.13  Fig. 4.14

## movement 5

**1.** Maintain rhythmic breathing as you lift your upper body to vertical, placing the hands on the front knee to support the weight of the upper body (fig. 4.9).
**2.** Inhale as you lift the hips off the ball, keeping the spine vertical. The back knee straightens slightly.
**3.** On the exhale engage the transverse abdominis as you lower the body to make contact with the ball again. The back knee bends slightly to accommodate the lunge position of the legs.

## movement 6

**1.** Inhale and raise the arms overhead, lightly pressing the palms together (fig. 4.10).
**2.** Exhale.
**3.** Inhale as you raise your hips off the ball (fig. 4.11). Continue to press the palms together lightly.
**4.** On an exhale engage the transverse abdominis as you lower the hips onto the ball, still extending the arms overhead.
**5.** Inhale.
**6.** On an exhale engage the transverse abdominis as you bend gently backward (fig. 4.12).
**7.** Take a full inhale.

## movement 7

**1.** Exhale, check your transverse abdominis activation, and release the backbend. Release the arms to your sides, maintaining a lunge position on the ball (fig. 4.13).
**2.** Lift your hips off the ball and roll the ball to your left side, then lower into a kneeling position (fig. 4.14).

## movement 8

Continue to breathe rhythmically as you bring the left leg back to join the right in a kneeling position behind the ball, both hands resting lightly on the top sides of the ball.

51

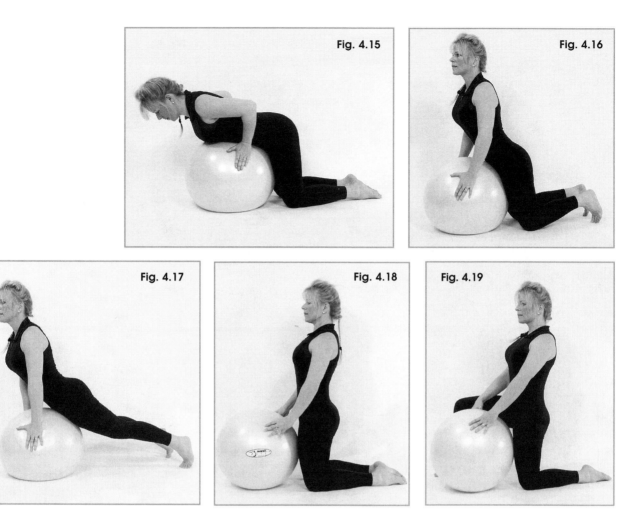

Fig. 4.15

Fig. 4.16

Fig. 4.17

Fig. 4.18

Fig. 4.19

### movement 9

**1.** On an exhale engage the transverse abdominis and lower your chest to the ball (fig. 4.15). This is Half Plank position.

**2.** Curl the toes under and inhale as you lift your chest from the ball, rising into a gentle backbend as you partially straighten the arms (fig. 4.16). This is beginner-level Cobra asana.

**3.** Exhale as you bend your arms and lower your chest to the ball. Check the activation of your transverse abdominis.

**4.** Breathe rhythmically as you roll the ball forward slightly and straighten the knees. Inhale as you press into a backbend, the advanced-level Cobra (fig. 4.17).

**5.** On an exhale release the Cobra, rolling

back down onto your knees (see fig. 4.16). Your arms support you on the ball.

### movement 10

**1.** Rise to a vertical kneeling position behind the ball, resting your hands lightly on the ball's surface (fig. 4.18).

**2.** Roll the ball to the left side of the body as you bring the right knee forward in line with the ball. Hands are placed on the top sides of the ball (fig. 4.19). You are now in an easy lunge position.

**3.** Lift the back (left) knee from the floor and slip the ball underneath your pelvis (fig. 4.20). You're now prepared to execute Sun Salutation on the other side.

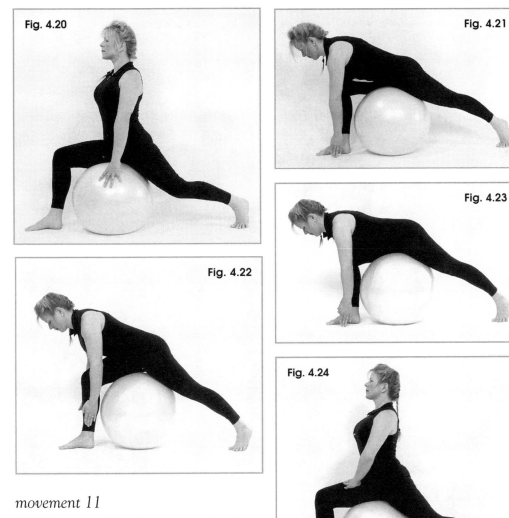

Fig. 4.20

Fig. 4.21

Fig. 4.22

Fig. 4.23

Fig. 4.24

## movement 11

**1.** Fold forward at the hips as you extend the left leg back, reaching the hands toward the floor on either side of the right foot (fig. 4.21).

2. Inhale as you straighten the back (left) knee, lifting the hips off the ball (fig. 4.22). The lower part of the back thigh maintains only slight contact with the ball. Feel the stretch in the left groin and the front of the left thigh.

**3.** On an exhale engage the transverse abdominis as you bend the back knee slightly and deepen the sink of the front thigh, taking care not to bend that knee past 45 degrees. The upper left thigh rests on the ball once again (fig. 4.23).

## movement 12

**1.** Maintain rhythmic breathing as you lift your upper body to vertical, placing your hands on your knee to support the weight of your upper body (fig. 4.24).

**2.** Inhale as you lift your hips off the ball. The back knee straightens slightly.

**3.** On the exhale engage the transverse abdominis as you lower the

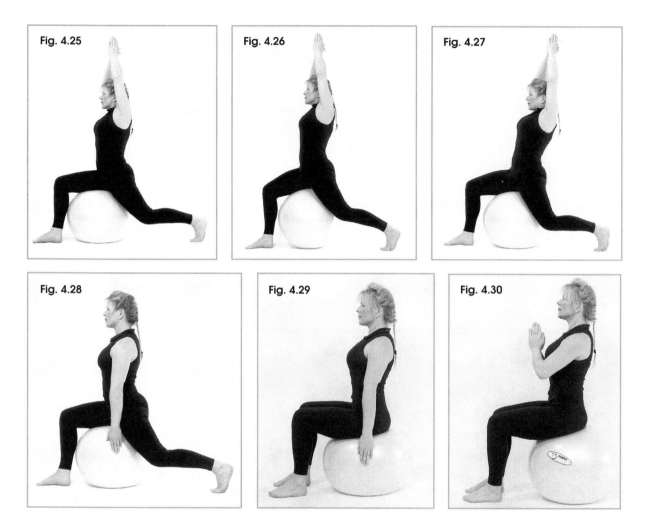

Fig. 4.25    Fig. 4.26    Fig. 4.27

Fig. 4.28    Fig. 4.29    Fig. 4.30

body to make contact with the ball again. The back knee bends slightly to accommodate the lunge position of the legs.

## movement 13

**1.** Inhale and raise the arms overhead, lightly pressing the palms together (fig. 4.25).
**2.** Exhale.
**3.** Inhale as you raise your hips off the ball (fig. 4.26). Continue to press the palms together lightly.

**4.** On an exhale engage the transverse abdominis as you lower the hips to the ball, still extending the arms overhead.
**5.** Inhale.
**6.** On an exhale engage the transverse abdominis as you bend gently backward (fig. 4.27).
**7.** Take a full inhale.

## movement 14

**1.** Exhale, check your transverse abdominis activation, and release the backbend. As you come to vertical release the arms and

bring them to your sides, maintaining your lunge position on the ball (fig. 4.28).
**2.** Bring the back leg forward to join the front so you are in a well-aligned seated position (fig. 4.29).

## movement 15

**1.** Bring the hands into prayer position in front of your chest (fig. 4.30).
**2.** Take two long, full diaphragmatic breaths here. Sit quietly and feel the heat rising in your body and your heart gently pumping blood to the extremities.

As you practice the Sun Salutation take note of anything that you observe that might give you useful information about the condition of your body. Did you feel excessive tension in any area of your body? If so, perhaps you need to spend more time warming that part with gentle and rhythmic range-of-motion movements, and in your cool-down lengthen the muscle fibers there with gentle stretchs. Were any areas of soreness or pain brought to your attention once you initiated movement? If so, observe these areas as you move through your yoga practice, being sure to journal your observations. If these problem areas persist consult your health care provider about them. The warm-up provides you with the opportunity to use present-moment awareness to tune in to your body; don't rush through. Schedule adequate time for a warm-up so you can be present to observe and absorb the information your body communicates to you in this essential phase of your practice.

The warm-up also prepares you psychologically for the work ahead. Beginnning a workout without mental preparation is similar to jumping out of bed and throwing your clothes on the second your feet hit the floor so you can get to work on time. All of us have experienced those times when we feel rushed, scattered, and unprepared for what lies ahead. A well-executed warm-up prevents your nervous system and your mood from being negatively impacted by being unprepared. Take your time. Observe the incremental changes in your breathing and heart-rate patterns that gradually prepare you for the activity to come.

The warm-up is the time to begin noticing how our breath patterns change and mold as we move through the basic postures of Surya Namaskar. Notice how your breathing patterns change as movement is introduced. If you notice that your breathing is labored or you feel as if you do not have enough breath to comfortably move through your warm-up, decrease your speed so that the breath can more easily accommodate your body's activity.

Act upon the information being communicated to you, adjusting your pace and your practice to fit your needs on any given day. Honor your body as you move into the heart of your practice.

# 5

# Yoga Asanas—
# Striking the Balance
# Between Strength
# and Flexibility

Practicing yoga asanas benefits so many aspects of our being. Yoga nourishes the mind by encouraging present-moment focus. If you are truly one-pointed in executing a posture and linking your breath with movement you cannot be thinking of anything else. In this way yoga asana practice helps to rid the mind of unnecessary chatter, giving you reprieve from everyday stressors as well as other challenges you may be facing in your life. The addition of the ball to yoga practice provides variety for your asana workout, helping to keep the mind stimulated. It also provides you with new opportunities for developing concentration and discipline.

As we've already discussed, yoga asana practice improves the health of the body in countless ways. Like many other forms of exercise yoga strengthens the muscles, ligaments, and joints. Yoga asana practice also improves the health of the organs and the adrenal and other endocrine glands. The exercise ball allows you to experience yoga postures in ways not possible on the mat alone. With the exercise ball as a partner some yoga postures will become more accessible to you; others will provide a unique challenge, given the unstable base that the ball provides. Working with the ball sharpens our proprioception, the body's sense of where it is in space at any given moment in time. We've not yet discussed this remarkable system. An athlete relies on her proprioceptors, sensory organs housed in the skin, muscles, and joints, to give her information that will make her efficient at her sport. Consider the mountain biker riding downhill who must negotiate challenging terrain so that she does not fall off her bike. Like any athlete that biker must constantly change her center of gravity to match the movements integral to her sport.

Proprioceptors provide information to the brain, which is then relayed to the muscles, so that a person can fine-tune his movements to address what is required of him spatially at any given moment. By introducing the element of mobility the ball encourages keenness in the body's proprioceptive sense.

The health of the spirit is also addressed through asana practice. Linking breath with movement balances the nervous system and helps us to relax into the moment. Contemplation and inner reflection come easier to us at these times. Executing yoga postures on the ball can be a movement meditation. The asanas in chapter 8 are designed to bring about deep relaxation. If deepening your spiritual sensibility is one of your goals in practicing yoga, these asanas will help you relax your body enough that you naturally move into spiritual thought and contemplation.

## Vinyasa—The Practice of Sequencing

In a hatha yoga practice the postures are sequenced specifically for optimum benefit to the body. The syllables that make up the word *hatha* are *ha*, meaning "sun," the masculine energy, and *tha*, "moon," the female energy. According to yogic theory every person has both energies present within; the practice of yoga unites these opposites and complements.

The organization of postures into a sequence is called *vinyasa*. In building a yoga practice each posture should either complement or counterbalance the previous one. For instance, one posture may extend only the upper part of the body; Cobra is a good example. The Cobra posture extends the back and stretches the chest. In asana practice Cobra would be followed by Locust, a complementary posture that extends the lower part of the body. Locust asana stretches the hip flexors and quadriceps and strengthens the gluteal muscles.

For optimal benefit to the body a counterbalancing posture, such as Forward Fold, would follow both of these asanas. A counterbalancing posture is one that engages the muscles opposite those you have just been using. In this example the back-bending series would be followed by a forward bend series. In other words, extension is followed by flexion, which is followed by extension again.

One of the outstanding benefits of the Yoga on the Ball sequence outlined in this chapter is that the exercises were carefully chosen to develop and maintain muscular balance throughout the entire body. As a fitness trainer and yoga teacher I am vigilant about this in my work with students. In Yoga on the Ball we sequence the postures to emphasize creating balance in the musculature given our twenty-first-century lifestyles.

Most people in our culture use the front of the body more than the back. Consider that when you push a shopping cart, lift and carry a bag of groceries, or open a car door you are training your pectoral (chest) muscles. When you climb stairs or even shift your legs under your desk you are training your quadriceps (thigh) muscles. For many the weak back muscles brought on by slouching over a desk or putting in lots of driving miles are paired with these tight chest muscles and quadriceps, along with tight hip flexors and hamstrings. Carrying the body with poor posture can also bring about muscular imbalance, as can your sport or preferred fitness activity.

The asanas in this chapter focus on strengthening muscles that are typically weak and creating flexibility in areas of the body that are most often tight. Flexibility needs are relative to the joint(s) being worked. To function optimally the body needs some muscles to be flexible whereas others need to be tighter in order to support the function of the joint. It is actually possible to have too much flexibility—in a situation like this the joint becomes hypermobile and thus vulnerable to injury. A delicate balance between strength and flexibility is needed for the body's optimal functioning. The functional workout trains the body for mobility and stability. We cannot sacrifice one for the other.

## The Asanas

For each asana in this chapter and the chapters that follow you will be given specific instruction regarding how to enter the pose, how to maintain the pose, and how to exit it safely. When you practice a posture on one side it needs to be repeated exactly the same way on the opposite side of the body in order to promote symmetry and balance. Pay careful attention to the instructions given for the use of the breath in each posture. Working with the breath and linking it with the movements involved in the asana are essential ingredients of any yoga practice. Many of my students have shared with me that their practice comes alive when they really begin to feel their movements inextricably linked with their inhales and exhales. Be patient with yourself here—it can take time to develop the skill of yoking your breath with your movement and lengthening the inhale and exhale to make that linking feel natural.

Before launching into the full practice of an asana I advise that you first spend time learning the mechanics of the pose. Practice it without being concerned about the breath and then, once you understand how the posture is to be executed, begin to link the breath with the movement. Approach the process of pairing breath with movement with a sense of fun and a willingness to play and experiment. Perfection is not the point; embodiment, fluidity, and the recognition that inspiration literally flows through us are the gifts of linking breath and movement in yoga.

In each day's yoga practice you want to find what the Buddha called the "middle way," the path between two extremes. Full expression of an asana is strong and steady, yet comfortable enough to not cause a reflexive tightening in parts of the body that are not being directly worked by the posture. Feel free to challenge yourself, to feel your muscles working hard and your joints opening, but at the point at which you feel anything more than moderate tension, back off a bit. If you press into a stretch beyond gentle tension you will actually cause the muscle that you are stretching to tighten rather than release, in order to protect itself from tearing. Refraining from harming yourself or others *(ahimsa)* is an essential part of the practice of yoga. There is no more immediate place to internalize this important tenet than moment to moment in the strong work of asana practice. Stay *sthira* (steady) and *sukha* (comfortable), letting prana flow through your body with each breath.

## Standing Forward Fold (Uttanasana)

In a traditional yoga practice the Forward Folds are usually practiced immediately after the preparatory pranayama (breathing) work and the Sun Salutation. Forward Fold is always followed by a counterbalancing asana, such as Cobra. Forward folds help to massage the internal organs by giving them a gentle kneading when the trunk moves toward the lower limbs. Blood is wrung out of the organs; the organs are then bathed with fresh oxygenated blood that flows in as the body opens after the forward-squeezing motion. Yogic theory tells us that Forward Folds decrease bloating and promote clear thinking.

When performing forward folds it is important to customize the fold to fit your individualized levels of strength and flexibility. If your forward bends go beyond 60 degrees of flexion you need to support yourself with a chair, against a wall, or with an exercise ball. Without that support you are literally hanging off the passive structures of the spine—the discs and ligaments—and this can cause damage to the spine. Properly executed forward folds can help strengthen your back, since the erector spinae muscles are required to pull you back up into extension. When practicing the Forward Fold bend only as far down as will allow you to maintain a neutral, well-aligned spine. If you are about to lose neutral spine you should not lower yourself any farther toward the floor, but rather stop where you are able to maintain correct alignment.

**Purpose** To strengthen the muscles of the back and stretch the hamstring muscles (the back of the thighs). This asana teaches the practitioner how to maintain neutral spine while performing folds.

**Watchpoints** • Maintain a lengthened spine throughout. • Do not flex the spine. • Keep the knees soft; make sure not to lock them. • Once you have found neutral spine, make sure to keep the retraction at the shoulder blades.

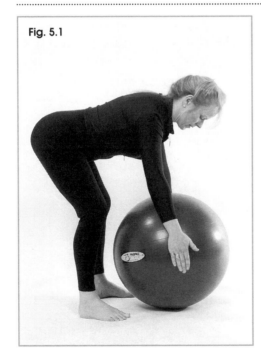

**Fig. 5.1**

*starting position*

Stand with your feet shoulder-distance apart and your knees slightly bent, the ball in front of you on the floor. Use Postural Setup to find neutral spine.

*movement*

**1.** On an exhale, gently engage the transverse abdominis.
**2.** Maintaining a lengthened spine, fold forward from the hips. Fold only as far as you can while maintaining neutral spine (fig. 5.1).
**3.** Hold this position for three full breaths.
**4.** Return to the starting position.
**5.** Repeat one more time. Notice whether you are able to fold farther in the second repetition.

# Seated Forward Fold

This asana provides a welcome stretch for the hamstrings. It is easier to limit the degree of flexion in the seated Forward Fold because the trunk is closer to the ground than it is in standing Forward Fold. Current exercise science suggests that the trunk be supported at flexion that exceeds 60 degrees to prevent damage to the spine. Where you are comfortable placing your hands—on the ball, on your knees or ankles, or on the floor—is directly related to the flexibility of your hamstrings. This placement of the hands provides a baseline for comparing how much the hamstrings lengthen through repeated practice.

**Purpose** To stretch the hamstring muscles. To strengthen the erector spinae, the muscles that run alongside the spine, and to massage the internal organs.

**Watchpoints** • Make sure to keep the back straight and the neck long. • Once you have found neutral spine be sure to keep the retraction at the shoulder blades.

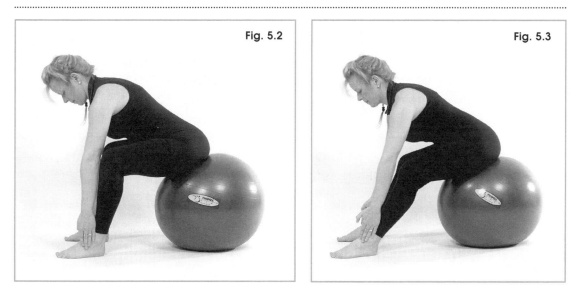

Fig. 5.2

Fig. 5.3

*starting position*

Sit tall on the ball, feet parallel and shoulder-distance apart. Use Postural Setup to find neutral spine.

*movement*

**1.** On an exhale gently engage the transverse abdominis and fold forward from the hip joint without flexing the spine (fig. 5.2). Place your hands on the ball, or on your knees, your ankles, or the floor to support your trunk.

**2.** Inhale as you roll the ball backward until you feel a gentle stretch in the hamstrings (fig. 5.3).

**4.** Exhale and gently engage the transverse abdominis again. Roll the ball forward.

**5.** Repeat two to three times.

# Cobra (Bhujangasana)

We follow the flexion of the forward bends with back extension, the movement essence of Cobra asana. Supported extension is most therapeutic for the back—this asana strengthens the erector spinae muscles, which extend the spine, and the rhomboids, the muscles that position the scapulae relative to the spine. By extending the back this asana also provides a strong stretch to the front of the body, expanding the rib cage and lengthening the muscles of the chest, including the muscles involved in breathing. This can be welcoming relief to those who deal with asthma. If you are to maintain proper muscle balance in the body in terms of the flexibility and strength ratio this posture is a must do.

One of the most common errors in executing this pose is overarching the back. If you experience a pinching sensation or any pain or discomfort in the back while executing this posture you are overarching. As you work with this pose try to remain cognizant of lengthening the spine at all times—visualize yourself creating space between each vertebrae with every breath you take. This focus will help to counteract any tendency to overarch. If you are a beginning exerciser or are new to yoga you may find that you rely on your arm muscles to lift your trunk rather than allowing the erector spinae to do their job of extending the back (and thus raising the chest). Avoid the temptation to use the arm muscles here; keep the extension low instead. As the back muscles strenghten you will be able to lift your upper body higher off the ball without the assistance of the arms. Progress to level two when you feel you have both the balance and strength necessary to be able to execute and maintain the posture for six seconds.

I find Cobra to be an exhilarating pose to execute. I practice it often when I am facing new challenges, reminding myself that I am opening to new opportunities and all that is good and available to me in the vast magnificence of this universe.

**Purpose** To help maintain proper alignment of the vertebrae. To strengthen the erector spinae muscles of the back, which extend the spine, and the rhomboids, the muscles between the spine and the shoulder blades that retract the shoulder blades. To stretch the muscles of the chest and the abdominals.

**Watchpoints** • Focus on the muscles of your back—rather than relying on your arm muscles—to lift your chest. • Keep the spine and neck lengthened at all times. Do not overarch the back; this can result in compression of the vertebrae, causing harm to the spine. • Keep the scapulae stabilized. • Maintain an active transverse abdominis throughout the entire movement.

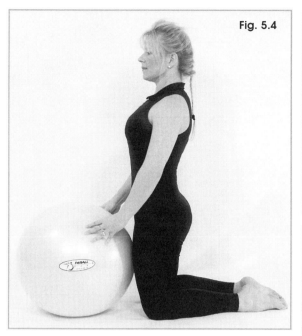

Fig. 5.4

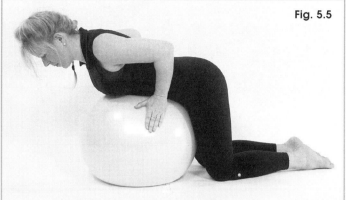

Fig. 5.5

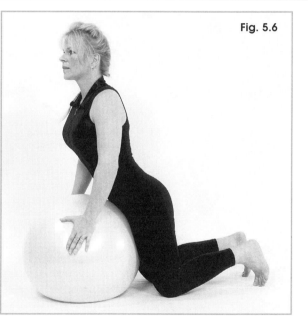

Fig. 5.6

## starting position

**1.** Kneel behind the ball and draw the ball in close to your body (fig. 5.4).

**2.** Drape yourself over the ball, resting your chest on the ball (fig. 5.5). Your hands are at the top sides of the ball.

## movement—level one

**1.** Lengthen the spine. On an exhale engage the transverse abdominis by gently drawing the navel toward the spine.

**2.** On the inhale engage the erector spinae muscles alongside the spine to slowly lift your upper body off the ball, arching into a back extension (fig. 5.6). The ball will roll slightly forward with this move. Knees remain in contact with the floor. If you feel pinching or pain in the back you are arching your spine too much.

**3.** Hold this posture for 6 seconds if you can. Remember to keep breathing. Try to work up to holding the pose and breathing for 1 minute.

**4.** Exhale as you lower your chest to the ball.

**5.** Repeat the asana three times.

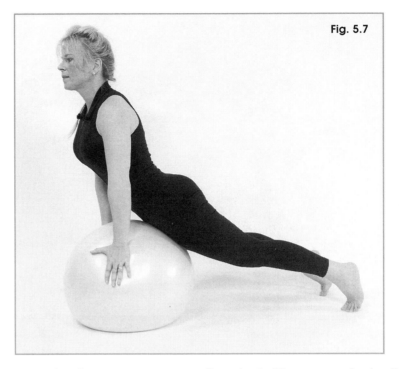

**Fig. 5.7**

*movement—level two*

**1.** Lengthen the spine. Kneel behind the ball and draw the ball close to the body (see fig. 5.4).

**2.** Drape yourself over the ball, resting your chest on the ball. Your hands are on the top sides of the ball (see fig. 5.5).

**3.** On an exhale engage the transverse abdominis by gently drawing the navel toward the spine.

**4.** Curl the toes under and press off the feet to roll the ball forward, straightening your knees as you simultaneously inhale and engage the muscles along the spine to lift your upper body off the ball (fig. 5.7). You're now arched in a gentle backbend, legs long and strong behind you. Resist your thigh muscles away from the floor without overtightening your buttocks.

**5.** Hold this posture for 6 seconds. Don't forget to keep breathing. Try to work up to holding the pose and breathing for one minute.

**6.** Exhale as you lower your chest to the ball.

**7.** Repeat three times.

# Down Dog (Adhomukha Svanasana)

Down Dog is the perfect counterbalance to Cobra. In this asana gravity provides traction for the elongation of the spine, taking pressure off the intervertebral discs and creating space between the vertebrae while maintaining the spine in a neutral position. Down Dog is an excellent posture for people who need to lengthen the spine to ease the pain associated with degenerative disc disease.

The most common training error in this pose is failing to stabilize the shoulder blades. It is easy to lose stabilization when you are in this inverted position because the shoulder blades want to drop toward your ears (that is, toward the ground) due to the effect of gravitational forces. For many people the shoulder blades are already in the undesirable protracted position as a result of daily activities—slouching over a desk, driving a car—that stretch rather than strengthen the scapular muscles. Engage the rhomboids, the muscles between the shoulder blades and the spine, to maintain a slight retraction of the shoulder blades. Use discipline and discernment to sense where your shoulder blades are at all times when executing Down Dog.

Moving in and out of this pose as well as maintaining the pose require using muscles of both the upper and lower body. Every time I practice this pose I am reminded that there is a delicate balance that needs to be maintained in life. Down Dog may show you to be strong, but if you are not flexible you may have some trouble initially negotiating this pose. On the other hand, if you are flexible but lack in strength you will not be able to hold the pose for very long. Regular practice of this asana develops the strength *and* the flexibility required to execute this pose properly. This pose reminds us that we are continually challenged to maintain a balance in our lives in terms of the energies we direct toward family, career, and the other things that are important to us. Overabundance in one area can lead to deficiency in other areas. It is important to be patient, to set our trajectories, and to move in the direction that seems most right in each moment.

**Purpose** To strengthen the chest, arm, and shoulder muscles, as well as the quadriceps (front of the thighs). To lengthen the spine through gravity-induced traction. To stretch the front of the shoulders (the deltoids), the back of the thighs (the hamstrings), the buttocks, and the calves.

**Watchpoints** • Keep the scapulae stabilized throughout the entire pose. • Maintain a slight bend in the knees and the elbows. Limit the anterior tilt of the pelvis if you lack flexibility in the hamstrings and calves. • Be careful not to press the upper body into the stretch too intensely if you have tight chest or shoulder muscles or have problems with your shoulder joint. • People with high blood pressure or glaucoma should not practice inverted poses without first consulting a physician.

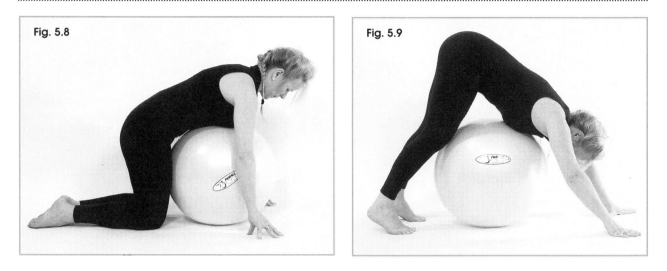

Fig. 5.8

Fig. 5.9

### starting position

Kneel behind the ball on your hands and knees, the ball positioned under your trunk to support your body weight (fig. 5.8). Your hands are lined up directly under the shoulder joints and knees are directly under the hip joints. Engage the rhomboid muscles to stabilize the shoulder blades.

### movement

**1.** On the exhale gently engage the transverse abdominis, curl the toes under, and lift the buttocks toward the ceiling so that the trunk and legs form an inverted V (fig. 5.9). Let the ball roll with your body to support the chest. Do not worry if your heels don't touch the floor.

**2.** Breathe rhythmically in this position, maintaining length through the spine. Do not flex or hyperextend the neck; rather, keep the head in line with the spine.

**3.** You may wish to alternately reach the heels toward the floor to increase the stretch in the calf muscles.

**4.** You can increase or decrease the intensity of the hamstring stretch in this pose. If you drop your hips slightly (the ball will roll toward your hands) you will decrease the stretch in the top of the hamstrings. If you lift your hips (the ball rolls slightly toward your feet) and reach your heels to the floor you will increase the tension in the hamstring muscles.

**5.** Attempt to hold the pose for 10 seconds to start. Work up to holding for 30 seconds or more, breathing rhythmically throughout the stretch.

**6.** Lower your belly to the ball on an exhale.

**7.** Perform up to three repetitions of Down Dog. Take note of the intense activation in the arm muscles as well as the stretch that occurs through the back as traction does its job in this asana.

# Reverse, or Inclined, Plank (Purvottanasana)

This asana is a good counterbalance to Down Dog. Whereas Down Dog strengthens the front shoulder muscles and the quadriceps, Reverse Plank tones the rear part of the shoulders and arm (particularly the posterior deltoid muscles) and stretches the chest. Reverse Plank is also very efficient at improving core stability. Kundalini yoga theorists tell us that this posture strengthens the kidneys.

This posture can be intimidating to the beginner. If you are new to yoga you may not have the strength to execute a full Plank; if this is the case follow the instructions provided for level one. I am reminded when practicing this posture that we need to accept where we are today while still embracing our dreams for tomorrow.

**Purpose** To strengthen the rear deltoid muscles and stretch the chest (the pectorals) and front shoulder muscles. To develop core stability.

**Watchpoints** • Keep the shoulder blades gently drawn together. • Distribute the body's weight evenly between the hands. • Throughout the posture keep your head in line with your spine, chin retracted. • Concentrate on maintaining the activation of the transverse abdominis to keep the ball from rolling. • Be careful not to hold the breath. • If you have a hernia in the digestive canal or you have an acute rotator cuff (shoulder joint) problem seek the counsel of your health care professional before practicing this pose.

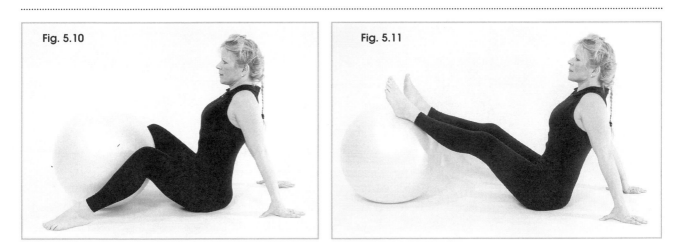

Fig. 5.10 Fig. 5.11

*starting position*

**1.** In a sitting position secure the ball between your feet. Place your hands behind your hips, fingers pointing away from the body (fig. 5.10).
**2.** Place one heel at a time on the top surface of the ball.
**3.** Balance at this point for one breath cycle (fig. 5.11).

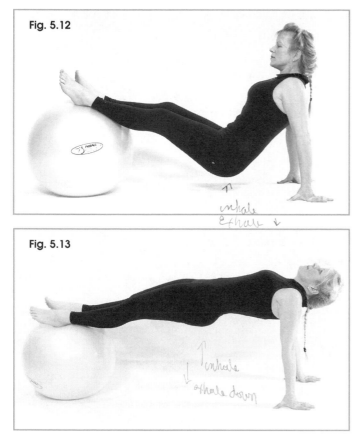

Fig. 5.12

Fig. 5.13

## movement—level one

**1.** On an exhale, engage the transverse abdominis by gently drawing the belly toward the spine.
**2.** Inhale as you lift the buttocks a few inches from the floor (fig. 5.12).
3. Attempt to hold the pose for 3 seconds, breathing rhythmically. Try to work up to holding the posture for 12 seconds.
**4.** Exhale, lowering the buttocks to the floor.
**5.** Repeat six to eight times, or move directly to level two.

## movement—level two

**1.** On an exhale engage the transverse abdominis, gently drawing the navel to the spine.
**2.** Inhale as you lift the buttocks from the floor until the body forms an unbroken plane (fig. 5.13).
**4.** Attempt to hold this posture for 3 seconds. Don't forget to breathe. Work up to holding the pose for 12 seconds.
**5.** Exhale, lowering the buttocks to the floor.
**6.** Perform six to eight repetitions.

# Camel Pose (Ustrasana)

The Camel is a complementary posture to the Plank due to the fact that it adds a backbend to the equation. This posture could be a staple in almost everyone's body-maintenance system because it opens the chest, extends the back, and tones core musculature, targeting areas that for most people need to be both stretched and strengthened.

Yogic theory holds that this posture stimulates the lungs and the heart. The abdominal stimulation imparted by this pose enhances functioning of the gastrointestinal system and decreases gas and constipation.

**Purpose** To strengthen the core muscles and tone the abdominals. To stretch the chest and the anterior shoulder muscles.

**Watchpoints** • Place a rolled towel under the knees if they are pained in this position. • Keep the scapulae stabilized. • Do not overarch the back. • Maintain transverse abdominis activation throughout the posture.

*starting position*

Rest on the knees and roll the ball around your body (fig. 5.14). Place the ball behind your body, between the ankles.

*movement*

**1.** On an exhale engage the transverse abdominis by gently drawing the navel to the spine and lean back just far enough so that you feel the abdominal muscles contracting to keep you in position (fig. 5.15).
**2.** Strive to hold this position for 12 seconds, breathing rhythmically.
**3.** Release the pose and roll the ball in front of you for a rest phase.
**4.** Perform Camel for a total of six to eight repetitions.

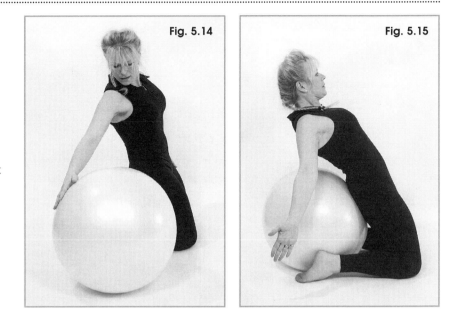

Fig. 5.14    Fig. 5.15

# Forward Fold with Spinal Twist (Prasarita Padottanasana 1)

This forward fold is an effective counterbalance to the Camel. Since the spine is warm now it is safe to introduce the spinal twist. The twist keeps the spine supple and is an excellent tension-releasing pose for people who work long hours and are prone to developing tightness and spasm in the back and shoulders. I find that the spinal twists "pump" tension out of my spine. Asanas that incorporate twists are also excellent for developing the stabilized yet free movement necessary for activities that involve rotation—especially if it is an instantaneous movement such as the rapid fire uncoiling of the golf swing.

It is imperative that this twist be executed slowly and thoughtfully. It is dangerous to perform *any* spinal twisting movement quickly. I often see spinal twists executed in the gym in a kind of ballistic fashion while the person holds on to a pole. This is a recipe for disaster—the vertebrae and discs must rotate perfectly and without fail to adequately protect the spine from being damaged. The controlled, gentle rotation presented in this asana is a more intelligent approach to stretching the rotators of the spine.

With the aid of a ball the Forward Fold with Spinal Twist is easy for most people to execute. The ball supports much of the body's weight, thereby decreasing the load on the upper extremities and the spine. Yogis believe that

69

forward folds create tapas (heat) in the body and help prana to circulate throughout the body. When I practice this pose I visualize the compression massage my organs receive as I flex into the forward bend.

**Purpose** To stretch the spinal rotators and recognize supported movement through the spine. To stretch the hamstrings and the muscles of the chest, especially the pectorals. To strengthen the upper body.

**Watchpoints** • Keep the neck and spine in a lengthened position. Do not bend the spinal column while twisting. • Avoid dropping the head. • Keep the scapulae stabilized. • Move slowly when twisting the spine.

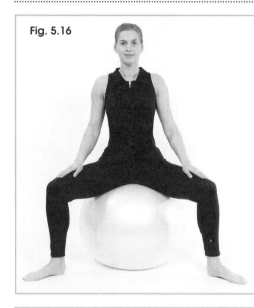

Fig. 5.16

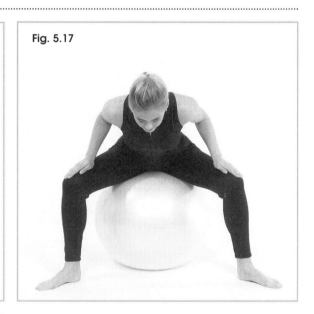

Fig. 5.17

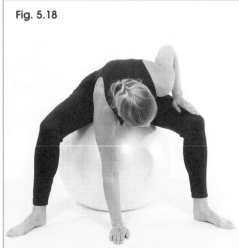

Fig. 5.18

*starting position*

Sit on the ball with your feet on either side of the ball, toes pointed outward, hands on the knees (fig. 5.16). Gently engage the rhomboid muscles to stabilize the shoulder blades.

*movement*

**1.** On an exhale engage the transverse abdominis by gently drawing the navel to the spine. Breathe rhythmically and diaphragmatically from this point to the end of the posture.
**2.** Fold forward from the hip joint while maintaining a straight back (fig. 5.17). The hands stay on the knees to support the weight of the upper body.
**3.** Place the right hand in the center of the space between your feet (fig. 5.18). Gently twist your

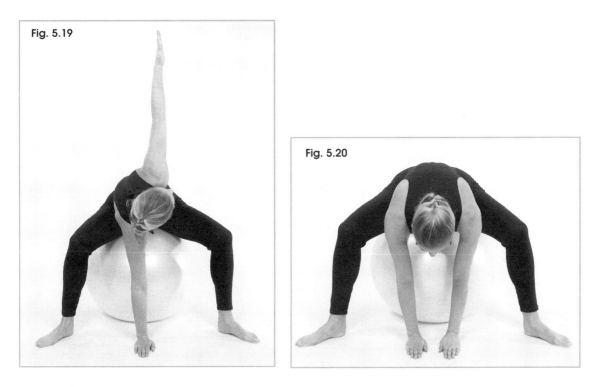

Fig. 5.19

Fig. 5.20

spine as you reach the left arm toward the ceiling, the palm facing away from the body (fig. 5.19). Create one long line from the fingertips of the lower arm to the fingertips of the top arm.

**4.** Look up. Concentrate on lengthening through the spine and positioning the top arm to fully open and stretch out the chest without torsioning through the hips.

**5.** Hold the posture for five full breaths.

**6.** Gently and slowly release the twist as you draw the top arm back toward the floor. Bring both hands to the floor in front of you (fig. 5.20).

**7.** Once you are balanced here, place the left hand on the floor at the midline of the body and execute the twist on the opposite side.

**8.** Perform at least two repetitions on each side of the body.

## Yoga Chair Pose (Uktatasana)

Chair Pose is a midrange spinal movement that returns the spine to a neutral position after a forward fold; it is an effective linking posture between a forward bend and a backward bend. In this posture the buttocks press out behind you as you lower your body toward the floor in a half squat. This is in no way a passive exercise—it requires that you actively use your back and legs to hold the position. Literally translated *Uktatasana* means "raised posture." Some yoga traditions refer to this as the lightning bolt pose, and if you look at a side profile of this posture you can see why.

If you lack flexibility in the shoulder joint you might find it difficult to hold your arms in alignment with your ears. Listen to what your body tells you. If it causes you discomfort to draw the arms that far back situate them so that you feel a gentle stretch in the shoulder with no discomfort.

Yoga theory states that this pose massages the heart and diaphragm. As I practice this pose I like to visualize that a mystical healing power housed in the heavens beams energy into my fingertips and is directed to whatever area of my body, mind, or spirit needs it on that particular day.

**Purpose** To strengthen the legs, buttocks, and the back of the arms. To stretch the latissimus dorsi, the widest muscle of the back. To return the spine to neutral position following the Forward Fold with Spinal Twist.

**Watchpoints** • Keep the neck long and the scapulae stabilized. • Ensure that the knees are lined up over the ankles in the "down" phase of the movement and that the knees do not press out over the toes.

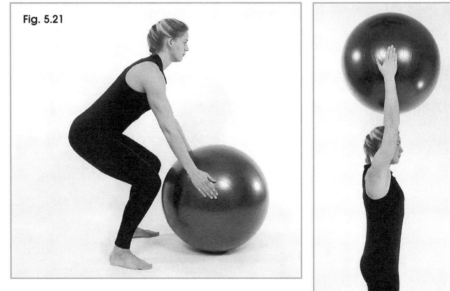

Fig. 5.21

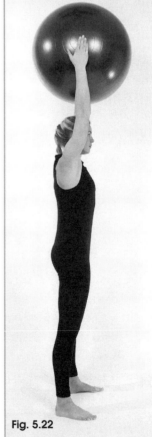

Fig. 5.22

*starting position*

**1.** Stand with your feet shoulder distance-apart and your knees slightly bent. Use Postural Setup to find neutral spine and a gentle retraction of the shoulder blades.
**2.** Bend the knees and squat to pick up the ball, maintaining a neutral spine (fig. 5.21).
**3.** With the ball secured between your palms extend your arms overhead, aligning your arms with your ears. Your shoulders, elbows, and hands create a straight line (fig. 5.22).

*movement*

**1.** On an exhale engage the transverse abdominis, then lower the buttocks toward the floor as you bend your elbows to lower the ball behind the head (fig. 5.23). Maintain the elbows and shoulders in a straight line and continue reaching the buttocks toward the floor until your knees are directly over your ankles.

**2.** Inhale as you straighten the arms and legs to come back to vertical (fig. 5.24).

**3.** Repeat six to eight times.

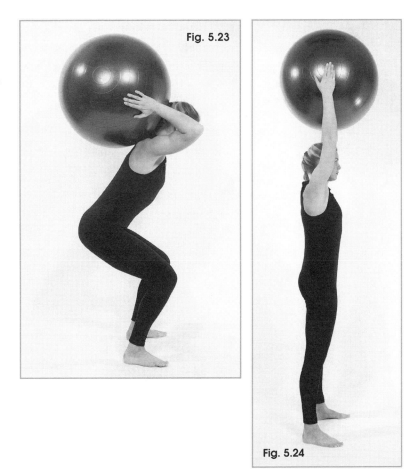

Fig. 5.23

Fig. 5.24

# Bow Pose (Dhanurasana)

This pose is a suitable counterbalance to any forward fold. This posture beautifully stretches the commonly overtight chest and extends the back, making it easier for the muscles involved in breathing to do their job. I particularly like this modified version of the Bow because the ball helps to prevent you from compressing the discs in the spine, which is often the mistake that yoga practitioners make when they yank at the ankles or hyperextend the back in this pose. This is also a superb posture for defining and lifting the gluteals.

People who lack strength in the back may find it difficult to raise the chest at first. Those who have weak gluteal muscles may have difficulty raising the legs off the floor. A lack of flexibility in the chest or hip flexor muscles (the psoas major, iliacus, and rectus femoris) can also create a challenge for moving into this posture. Being patient and practicing regularly will pay its dividends, and gradually the posture will become easier to execute.

73

I enjoy working with the image of the Bow. I like to think that when I treat my body to performing this revitalizing pose I am generating vital energy, just as the cord of the bow does before it releases the arrow. I then imagine myself storing the energy of the pose in my body so that it can be released at a later date, when I need to direct my vitality toward a predetermined goal.

**Purpose** To stretch the chest, the front of the thighs, and the deep psoas muscles; to strengthen and tone the back of the upper thighs, the buttocks, and the back.

**Watchpoints** • Keep the neck long. • Maintain scapular stabilization. • Do not overarch the back. • Maintain transverse abdominis activation through-

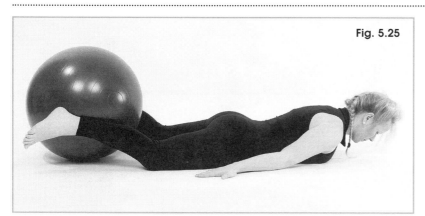

Fig. 5.25

out the movement.

*starting position*

Lie on your belly with the ball between the ankles. Arms are at your sides, palms down (fig. 5.25). Gently engage the rhomboid muscles to stabilize the shoulder blades.

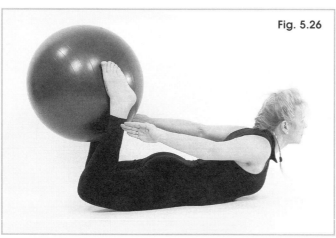

Fig. 5.26

*movement*

**1.** On an exhale engage the transverse abdominis by gently drawing the navel up and in toward the spine.
**2.** Breathe rhythmically as you simultaneously lift the upper body from the floor and bend the knees, bringing the ball close to the buttocks. Allow the arms to lift with the upper body into a gentle backbend, palms facing out (fig. 5.26). Press the heels toward the ceiling as you lift the upper thigh from the floor.
**3.** Hold for 6 seconds.
**4.** Lower the upper body, arms, and upper thighs to the floor.
**5.** Repeat six to eight times.

# Crow Pose (Kakasana)

The hip folding involved in this stretch is a good counterbalance to the work of the Bow pose. This posture provides a wonderful release in the hip and buttock area and I have therefore always found this to be a relaxing posture to sink into. You can control the intensity of the stretch by simply monitoring the roll of the ball—rolling the ball forward and dropping closer to the ground increases the stretch. This posture is thought to rid the body of lethargy. It helps relieve tension and soreness in the buttocks when you have been sitting for any significant length of time.

**Purpose** To stretch the buttocks and strengthen the thighs.

**Watchpoints** • Make sure that the knees are aligned over the ankles throughout the posture. • Maintain a gentle retraction through the shoulder blades.

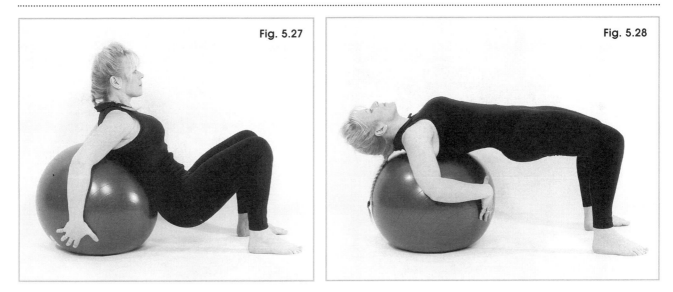

Fig. 5.27

Fig. 5.28

*starting position*

**1.** Sit in the center of your ball with your feet shoulder-distance apart. Use Postural Setup to find neutral spine and a gentle retraction of the shoulder blades.
**2.** Walk your feet out and then bend the hips and knees to sink down toward the floor (fig. 5.27). Your feet should be flat on the ground and pointed forward. The buttocks are two to three inches off the floor; arms hug the sides of the ball.

*movement—level one*

**1.** On an exhale engage the transverse abdominis.
**2.** Inhale, lifting your body into a tabletop position, the front of your body from your head to your knees in an unbroken plane (fig. 5.28). As you lift into tabletop the ball will roll toward the head. Keep your hands in place on the ball. Once you're in tabletop position readjust your arms for comfort if necessary. Make a nice straight line from head to knee.

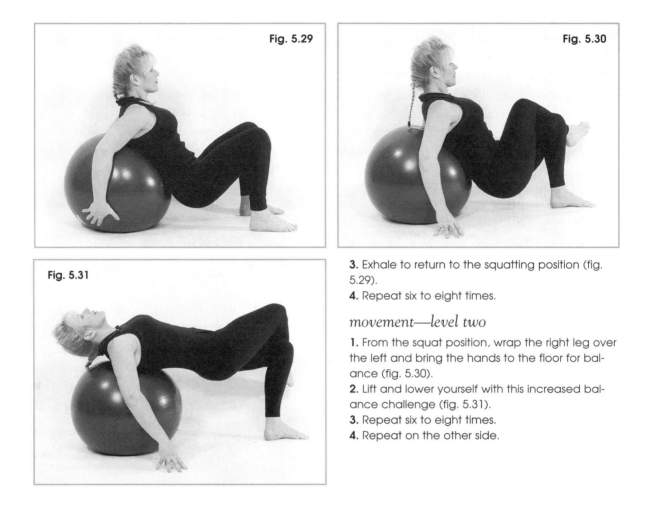

**3.** Exhale to return to the squatting position (fig. 5.29).
**4.** Repeat six to eight times.

*movement—level two*

**1.** From the squat position, wrap the right leg over the left and bring the hands to the floor for balance (fig. 5.30).
**2.** Lift and lower yourself with this increased balance challenge (fig. 5.31).
**3.** Repeat six to eight times.
**4.** Repeat on the other side.

## Modified Locust Pose (Salabhasana)

Locusts (grasshoppers) lift their hind ends up and down. When you practice this pose be mindful that you do not hyperextend the low back. As the hips raise you will want to bring your attention to the low back and buttocks—if you feel any pain or pinching in that area lower the hips toward the floor. As with the Bow pose, this asana is a wonderful pose for strengthening and toning the gluteal muscles.

Locust pose is said to improve digestion and elimination due to the increase in yogic digestive fire that is stimulated by the massage to the internal organs. When I practice this pose I visualize the strong legs that the grasshopper must have in order to propel himself from place to place, and I imagine the strength that my own body develops from performing this pose regularly.

**Purpose** To stretch the front of the thighs; to strengthen and tone the buttocks and the back of the thighs.

**Watchpoints** • Keep the neck long. • Stabilize the shoulder blades. • Do not overarch the low back. If you feel any pinching or tightening in the back make incremental adjustments in the hips, bringing them a bit closer to the floor.

*starting position*

**1.** Lying on your belly with knees bent at a 90-degree angle, secure the ball between the ankles (fig. 5.32).
**2.** Place one hand over the other and rest your chin on your hands.

*movement*

**1.** On an exhale engage the transverse abdominis. Squeeze the buttock muscles and lift the thighs slightly off the floor (fig. 5.33).
**2.** Breathe as you hold this position for 3 seconds.
**3.** Inhale as you release to the starting position.
**4.** Repeat six to eight times.

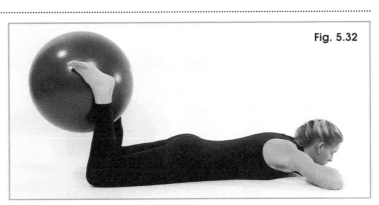

Fig. 5.32

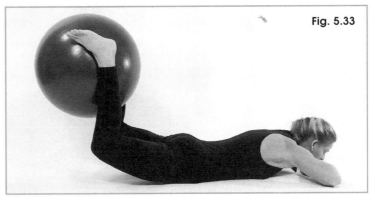

Fig. 5.33

# Side Plank or Arm Balance (Vashishthasana)

This is an effective pose to place at this point in your practice because it provides effective counterbalancing work. Side Plank works the upper body; it also complements the Locust by toning the muscles of the outer thigh. This asana is extremely useful for developing core stability and all-around upper body strength. People involved in skulling, kayaking, and other rowing sports find this posture beneficial to their training. If you do not have adequate strength in the stabilizing muscles of the shoulder girdle you won't be able to balance in this posture for long, but do persevere. This posture is great for toning and strengthening these small albeit most important muscles. Side Plank challenges a host of muscles: the triceps, shoulder stabilizers, pectorals, trapezius, lattisimus dorsi, hip abductors, ankle evertors, and iliotibial band. The additional movement pattern described here helps to tone the outer thigh.

It is easy to see how this posture got its name. When practiced properly the body forms an unbroken plane from head to toe that resembles a plank. The weight of the body is balanced on the arm. Yogic benefits derived from this posture are increased concentration and nonattachment. For me this posture takes a great deal of intention and determination to execute properly. I feel that by practicing it regularly I strengthen my ability to focus and my sense of self-direction.

**Purpose** To strengthen the core musculature. To strengthen the arms and shoulders. The movement variation allows you to tone your outer thighs at the same time that you challenge your core.

**Watchpoints** • Maintain scapular stabilization and keep the shoulders down and away from the ears. • Maintain length through the neck. Do not let the head drop. • As you position your body in one long, straight line from the tip of your head to your toes do not let the hip sag. • Actively utilize your core muscles to maintain balance.

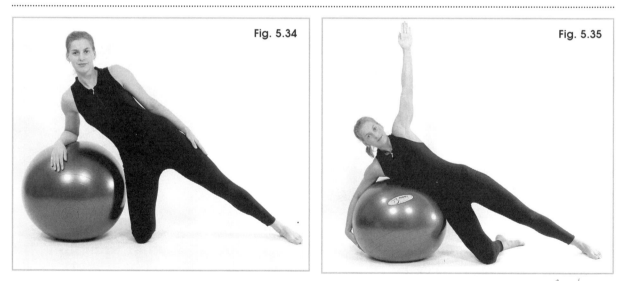

Fig. 5.34 / Fig. 5.35

*starting position*

1. Kneel with the ball positioned on your right side. Engage your rhomboid muscles to stabilize the scapulae.
2. Extend the left leg out to the side, resting your right arm on the top of the ball and the left arm on your left thigh (fig. 5.34).

*movement—level one* Exhale

1. Exhale as you engage the transverse abdominis and drape your right side over the ball, your right arm sliding down the ball and your left arm reaching toward the ceiling. Create a straight line from the shoulder joint to the fingertips (fig. 5.35). The fingers point toward the ceiling.

78

*Exhale Arm up*
*Inhale Arm rest on leg*
*Exhale leg up*
*Inhale lower leg.*

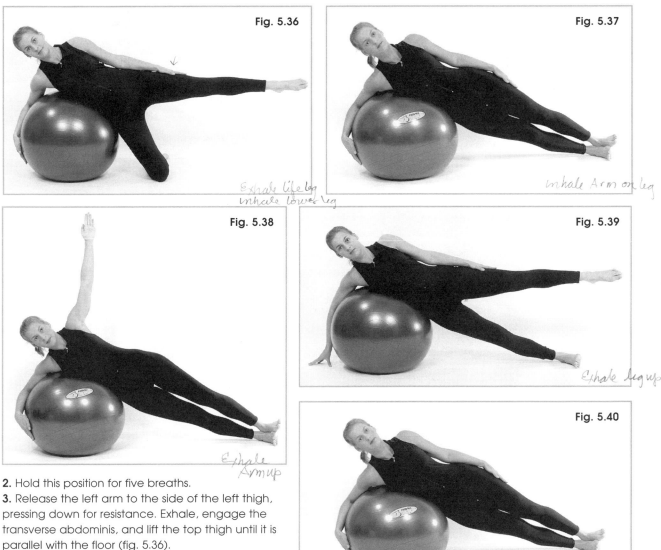

Fig. 5.36

*Exhale life leg*
*Inhale lower leg*

Fig. 5.37

*Inhale Arm on leg*

Fig. 5.38

*Exhale Arm up*

Fig. 5.39

*Exhale leg up*

Fig. 5.40

*Inhale leg down*

**2.** Hold this position for five breaths.

**3.** Release the left arm to the side of the left thigh, pressing down for resistance. Exhale, engage the transverse abdominis, and lift the top thigh until it is parallel with the floor (fig. 5.36).

**4.** Inhale as you lower the leg.

**5.** Repeat six to eight times, then switch to the left side by lowering yourself into a kneeling position and rolling the ball around to that side.

## movement—level two

**1.** Begin by draping your body sideways over the ball. Extend both legs long and align the ankle and hip of the top leg with the ankle and hip of the bottom leg. The left arm rests lightly on the upper thigh (fig. 5.37). Inhale.

**2.** Exhale and engage the transverse abdominis as you reach your top arm toward the ceiling, creat-ing a straight line from the shoulder joint to the fingertips (fig. 5.38). Fingertips reach toward the ceiling.

**3.** Hold for five breaths.

**4.** Release the arm to the side of the top thigh, pressing down to add resistance to the movement.

**5.** Exhale and lift the top thigh parallel to the floor (fig. 5.39).

**6.** Lower the left leg to rest on top of the right leg (fig. 5.40).

**7.** Repeat six to eight times, then switch to the other side by moving into a kneeling position and rolling the ball around to that side.

# Boat Pose (*Paripurna Navasana*)

Boat pose furthers the work of strengthening the core musclulature and toning the transverse abdominis. The core musculature is called upon in this asana to stabilize the spine while the body is challenged to hold the legs in a position unsupported by the floor or the ball. I have included several different levels of difficulty here—it is imperative that you determine which level is right for you. In level one you are instructed to raise your feet off the ball. Level two directs you to change your foot placement as well as your arm placement, intensifying the pose by changing your center of balance. Tremendous challenge is created in level three as you raise both the ball and the arms off the floor, significantly increasing the demands on the stabilizing musculature of the body. You will want to be careful that the movement level you choose as a starting point enables you to hold your spine in neutral position without the back being yanked into an excessive arch—which can be damaging to the spine—when you raise your legs.

According to yogic theory, Boat pose is thought to stimulate the kidneys, thyroid, prostate gland, and intestines. It also improves digestion.

**Purpose** To strengthen the core muscles and flatten the abdominals.

**Watchpoints** • Be sure not to round the back. • Be careful not to arch the back when you lift the feet from the floor. •Maintain transverse abdominis activation throughout the posture. • Do not practice this asana if you have high blood pressure, heart disease, or glaucoma.

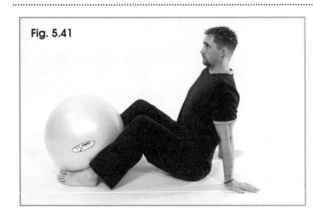

*starting position*

Begin in a seated position on the floor, knees bent and feet flat on the ground. Secure the ball between the feet. Hands are placed at the sides of the body behind the buttocks (fig. 5.41).

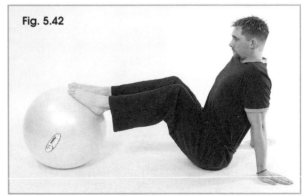

*movement—level one*

1. Lean back and shift your weight to your arms and upper buttocks as you place the soles of your feet on the top of the ball (fig. 5.42). Align your spine in ideal posture.

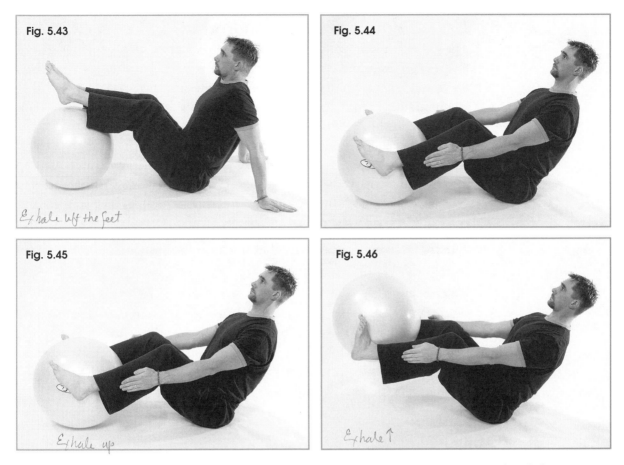

Fig. 5.43
Exhale off the feet

Fig. 5.44

Fig. 5.45
Exhale up

Fig. 5.46
Exhale ↑

**2.** Exhale and engage the transverse abdominis. Retract your chin and externally rotate your arms a bit. Inhale a full breath.
**3.** Check your transverse abdominis activation. Exhale as you lift the feet an inch off the ball (fig. 5.43).
**4.** Hold for six seconds, breathing rhythmically.
**5.** Release by lowering the feet to the ball.
**6.** Repeat two more times.

*movement—level two*

**1.** From the same starting position, exhale as you engage the transverse abdominis and raise the feet so that they grip the ball midway. Once you find your balance raise your arms so that they are in line with your feet (fig. 5.44).
**2.** Hold for six seconds. Make sure that you do not hold the breath but rather breathe smoothly and comfortably.
**3.** Release by lowering the arms to the side and relaxing the grip on the ball.
**4.** Repeat two more times.

*movement—level three*

**1.** Begin in the seated position with feet gripping midway on the outer sides of the ball, arms lined up nearly parallel with the lower legs (fig. 5.45).
**2.** Exhale, as you engage the transverse abdominis and lift the ball off the floor so that the ankles are almost parallel to the knees (fig. 5.46).
**3.** Attempt to hold for six seconds. Try to keep the breath rhythm smooth.
**4.** Release by lowering the arms and relaxing the grip on the ball.
**5.** Repeat two more times.

# Bridge Pose (Sethu Bhandasana)

The hip extension involved in Bridge pose provides a simple counterbalance to the hip flexion in Boat pose. Bridge pose is an effective toner for the buttocks and hamstrings and is useful for people who take part in sports that require training of the "push-off" musculature of the gluteals, responsible for propelling the body forward in an upright position.

Yogic benefits of this pose are thought to be increased circulation of blood and nutrients to the pituitary, thyroid, and adrenal glands. When you press up into this pose your body weight should be distributed between your feet and your upper back and shoulder blades: you should not feel that you are supporting your body weight in the neck area.

**Purpose** To strengthen and tone the muscles of the torso, the gluteals, and the hamstrings.

**Watchpoints** Keep your kneecaps facing toward the ceiling throughout the movement. • Maintain scapular stabilization. • Maintain a straight line from shoulders to buttocks to heels in the "up phase" of this asana. • Engage the transverse abdominis by drawing navel to spine. Fully utilize this core musculature to keep the ball steady. • Relax the neck. Position yourself so that you are not supporting your body weight in the neck area.

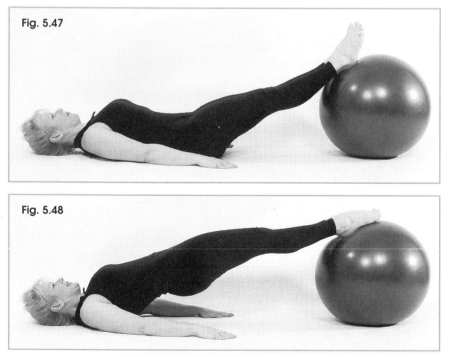

Fig. 5.47

Fig. 5.48

*starting position*

**1.** Lie on your back with your heels on the top surface of the ball (fig. 5.47). Gently draw the shoulder blades toward the spine. Make sure that the neck is long and shoulders are drawn down away from the ears.
**2.** Inhale.

*movement—level one*

**1.** On an exhale engage the transverse abdominis. Lift the buttocks off the floor until they are lined up with the heels, the body forming a straight line from the head to the feet (fig. 5.48).
**2.** Hold for two breaths.
**3.** Repeat six times at level one or move on to level two.

## movement—level two

**1.** Lie on your back with the soles of your feet resting on the surface of the ball (fig. 5.49). Your knees are directly above the hip joint, forming a 90-degree angle. Hands are resting at your sides.

**2.** Gently draw the shoulder blades toward the spine. Make sure that the neck is long and the shoulders are drawn down away from the ears.

**3.** Inhale.

**4.** On an exhale engage the transverse abdominis.

**5.** Lift the buttocks from the floor until they line up with the soles of the feet (fig. 5.50).

**6.** Roll the ball away from the body by straightening the legs, bringing the shoulders, buttocks, and heels into a straight line (fig. 5.51). Utilize the core muscles to maintain control of the ball. Do not lock the knees, and do not let the buttocks droop.

**7.** Roll the ball back toward your body (fig. 5.52).

**8.** Repeat the exercise six to eight times.

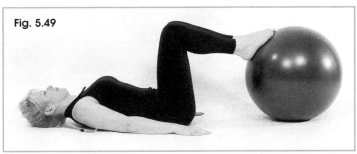

Fig. 5.49

*inhale prepare*

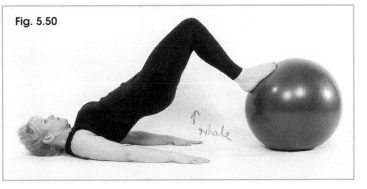

Fig. 5.50

*exhale*

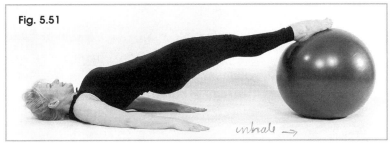

Fig. 5.51

*inhale →*

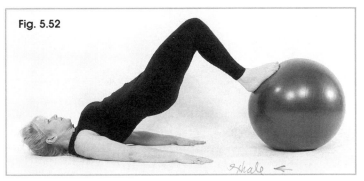

Fig. 5.52

*exhale ←*

# Warrior 1 (Virabhadrasana 1)

This asana provides a good counterbalance to the Bridge by changing the focus from the strengthening of the hamstring muscles to the stretching and strengthening of the reciprocal musculature, the quadriceps. In addition to being an effective toner for the thighs, Warrior pose provides a good stretch for the hip flexor muscles (the iliacus, psoas, and rectus femoris), which for most people are tight from frequent sitting. This posture also stretches the latissimus dorsi, the largest muscle of the back.

The Sanskrit root word for *virabhadrasana* can be translated as "hero." *Bhadra* means of "good omen." I am struck by the beauty of the body in this position, the arms reaching skyward to embrace the heavens while the feet remain firmly planted on Mother Earth. I interpret the placement of the arms in this posture to be a salute to the heavens, which to me symbolizes that the practitioner is seeking counsel from spirit above to learn how to carry on his or her duties here on Earth in the most noble and wise fashion possible.

**Purpose** To strengthen the quadricep muscles of the front leg. To stretch the quadriceps and hip flexor muscles of the back leg. To tone the stabilizing muscles of the inner thigh in both legs.

**Watchpoints** • Maintain scapular stabilization. • Maintain length through the neck and back. • Keep the knees aligned with the ankles, pevis in neutral alignment. If you begin to lose ideal form, stop. Increase your number of repetitions as you get stronger.

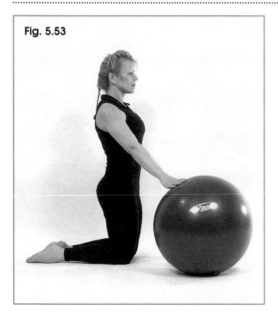

**Fig. 5.53**

*starting position*

Kneel with the ball in front of you, arms resting lightly on the ball. Engage the rhomboid muscles to gently draw the shoulder blades toward the spine, stabilizing the scapulae (fig. 5.53).

*movement—level one*

**1.** Exhale and engage the transverse abdominis. Bring your left knee forward into a lunge position (fig. 5.54). The ball is to the right of center.
**2.** Raise the ball overhead as you lift out of the lunge (figs. 5.55, 5.56, and 5.57). Make sure not to overarch the spine.
**3.** Release the ball to your right side and return to the lunge position (see fig. 5.54).
**4.** Return to the start position (see fig. 5.53) and execute on the opposite side.
**5.** Repeat eight to fifteen times, depending on your comfort level.

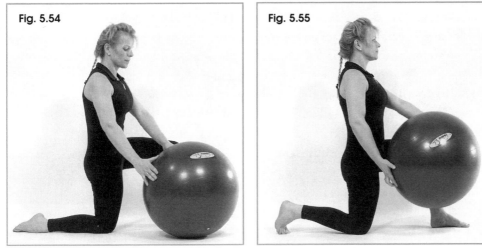

Fig. 5.54

Fig. 5.55

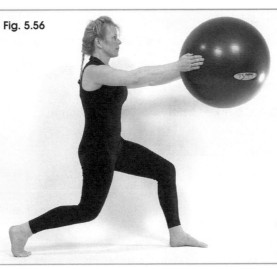

Fig. 5.56

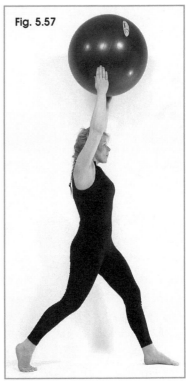

Fig. 5.57

## movement—level two

**1.** Begin in lunge position with the back knee raised from the floor. The ball is lifted off the floor and positioned in front of the right thigh (fig. 5.58).

**2.** On an exhale engage the transverse abdominis and raise the ball overhead with both hands as you raise yourself from the floor (see figs. 5.56 and 5.57). Inhale as you rise.

**3.** Exhale and lower the ball in front of your body (see fig. 5.58). Touch the ball to the midpoint of your knee as your knee lowers to the floor.

**4.** Repeat six to eight times.

**5.** Repeat on the other side of the body.

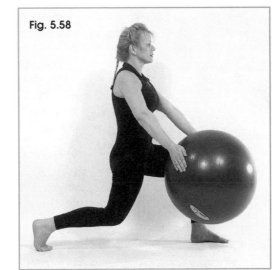

Fig. 5.58

85

# Warrior 2 (Virabhadrasana 2)

I view Warrior 2 as a progression of Warrior 1. The benefits of this posture are very similar to Warrior 1. Lifting and lowering your body in the Warrior position tones the quadriceps, gluteals, and hamstrings. This posture is useful for athletes who need to strengthen the quadriceps and stretch the inner thigh. It is also a good all-around strengthening pose for a beginning yoga practitioner because it trains a number of different muscle groups at once.

The Warrior 1 posture symbolizes to me that the practitioner is seeking counsel from the heavens to know how to approach his duties. In Warrior 2 the posture denotes to me that the practitioner has the answers he needs and is honing the skills needed to approach the challenge effectively. Practicing this posture can help to draw out and reinforce the admirable qualities of the warrior within you—inner strength, courage, and integrity. I have found this posture useful for helping me to connect with my inner strength, and I am left with a sense of grounded empowerment after practicing it.

**Purpose** To strengthen the quadriceps, gluteals, and hamstrings. To stretch the inner thigh.

**Watchpoints** • Maintain scapular stabilization. • Maintain length through the neck and back. • Be sure that the knee stays in line with the ankle.

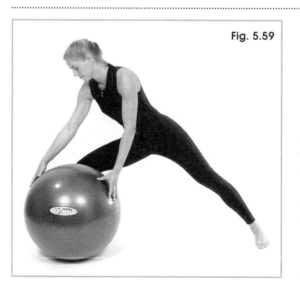

Fig. 5.59

### starting position

**1.** Begin in a strong standing position with the feet wide (three to four feet) apart. Turn the right foot 45 degrees outward; position the left foot so that the toes point in the same direction as the hips. You should be able to envision a straight line connecting the heel of your right foot with the arch of your left foot. The ball is on the floor by your right knee (fig. 5.59).
**2.** Place the ball on your right knee and sink into a lunge. The right knee is over the right ankle; there is a 90-degree angle between the shin and the back of the thigh. The right arm is long across the ball; the left arm is on the thigh (fig. 5.60).

### movement

**1.** On an exhale engage the transverse abdominis. Press your right arm down on the ball to create resistance as you elongate through the spine and deepen into the lunge. At the same

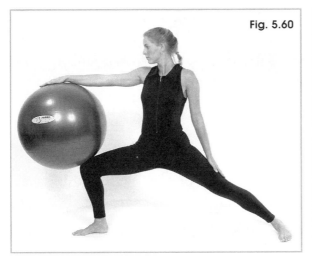

Fig. 5.60

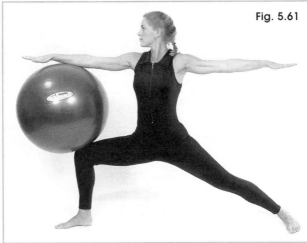

Fig. 5.61

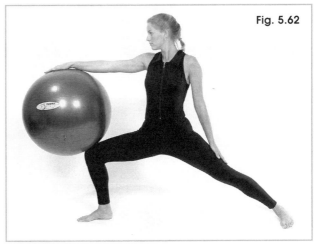

Fig. 5.62

time raise your left arm to create a straight line from fingertips to fingertips (fig. 5.61).

**2.** Inhale as you release the left arm and relax the lunge slightly (fig. 5.62).

**3.** Repeat six to eight times.

**4.** Return to the starting position and change sides: turn the left foot 45 degrees outward; position the right foot so that the toes point in the same direction as the hips. Envision a straight line connecting the heel of your left foot with the arch of your right foot. Place the ball on your left knee and sink into a lunge. The left knee is over the left ankle; notice the 90-degree angle between the shin and the back of the thigh. The left arm is long across the ball; the right arm is on the thigh.

**5.** Repeat Warrior 2 on the left side of the body.

## Extended Side Angle (*Parshvakonasana*)

Parshvakonasana gets its name from the *kona*, or angle, that the posture forms. This long, reaching asana provides a strong stretch for the oblique abdominals and other muscles that wrap around the side of the body, providing a fitting balance to the many forward and backward bends of a traditional yoga practice. When practicing this pose bring your attention to creating one long yogic line that extends from your heel to your fingertips. Actively use your muscles to reach through the fingertips, feeling the energy of the pose radiate through the fingertips. This maximizes the stretch through the oblique abdominals.

**Purpose** To stretch the muscles that wrap around the side of the body. To strengthen the quadriceps and the inner thigh.

**Watchpoints** • Make sure to stabilize the scapula by engaging the rhomboid muscles. • Maintain a straight spine throughout the asana.

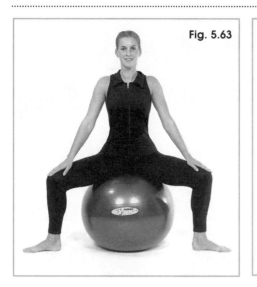

Fig. 5.63

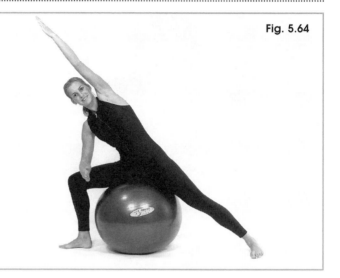

Fig. 5.64

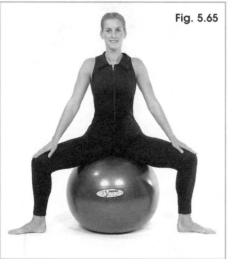

Fig. 5.65

*starting position*

Straddle the ball with legs wide, toes pointed out to sides. The arms rest lightly on the knees (fig. 5.63).

*movement*

**1.** Maintain the position of the right foot, toes pointing to the right. Rotate the left foot so that the toes point forward.
**2.** Exhale and engage the transverse abdominis. Extend the left hip to the left as you lean your upper body to the right, extending the left arm overhead and placing the right arm on the knee to support the upper body (fig. 5.64). You should feel one long, unbroken line extending from the heel of the left foot to the fingertips of the left hand. The fingers are long and straight.
**3.** Enjoy five diaphragmatic breaths as you fill out the shape of this asana, reaching long and strong through the fingertips.
**4.** Lower your arms to your thighs and raise your trunk so that the body weight is centered over the center of the ball. Return to the start position (fig. 5.65).
**5.** Rotate your left leg outward so that the toes point to the left. Rotate the right foot so that the toes point forward.
**6.** Repeat the posture on the left side.

# Warrior 1 with Prayer Twist

This variation of Warrior 1 offers the practitioner a gentle spinal rotation. All spinal rotations help eliminate tension from the spine and promote mobility and suppleness through the spine and the surrounding musculature. This spinal twist is a relaxing way to wind down your practice. As with any spinal twist, move slowly and carefully with control.

**Purpose** To release tension from the spine and promote spinal mobility.

**Watchpoint** • As with all spinal rotations, execute this pose slowly and with great attention to the alignment of the vertebrae.

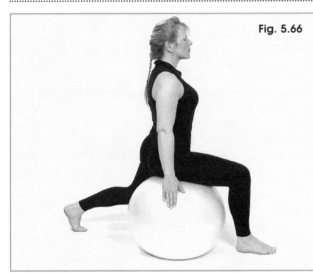

Fig. 5.66

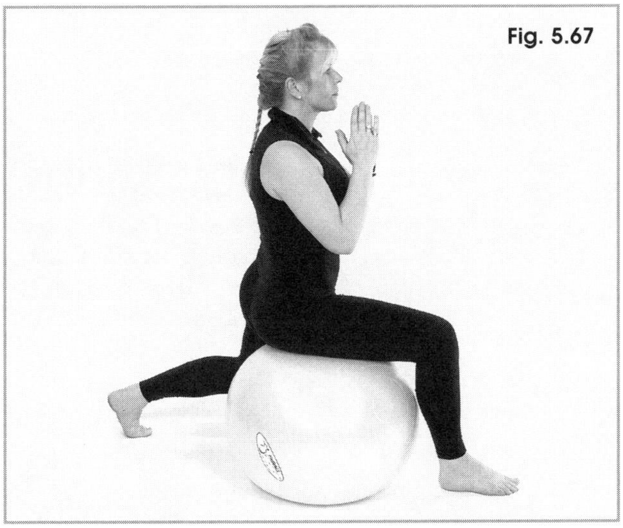

Fig. 5.67

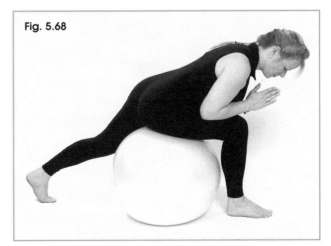

Fig. 5.68

*starting position*

Begin in lunge position on the ball, right leg forward (fig. 5.66).

*movement*

**1.** On an exhale engage the transverse abdominis. Breathe rhythmically.
**2.** Place the hands in prayer position at the breastbone (fig. 5.67). Inhale.
**3.** Exhale as you lower your upper body toward the right thigh, maintaining ideal alignment through the spine (fig. 5.68).

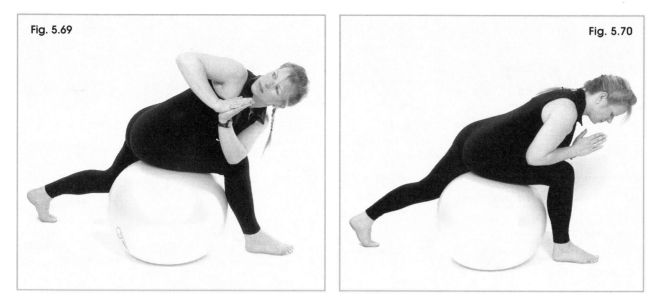

Fig. 5.69

Fig. 5.70

**4.** Beginning at the base of the spine, slowly rotate the trunk to the right (fig. 5.69). With each inhale lengthen through the spine; with each exhale deepen the rotation. The neck and head will be the last to turn.

**5.** Hold the rotation for five breaths, then slowly release your spinal twist (fig. 5.70). Lift the trunk to come into seated neutral position.

**6.** Repeat the asana with the left leg forward, rotating the trunk to the left.

As you become familiar with the idiosyncrasies of your body you will understand better how to fully utilize the asanas presented in this chapter to create that important balance between strength and flexibility.

Take your time with the process of getting to know your body. Use the feedback you receive in your asana practice to glean information necessary to make determinations about the relative strength and flexibility of various muscle groups. You deserve to live in a strong and balanced body. Know that both your body and your mind will benefit from yoga practice and this kind of information gathering, but the reaping of these rewards can only come through time, patience, and careful observation of what is specific to your body. Therefore, carefully consider the activities you take part in: what type of stretching and strengthening work is dictated by the activities of your life in order to create balance throughout your body? You might also want to examine the innate strengths, deficiencies, and areas of inflexibility with which you came into this life. And remember, if you are like most of us in the Western world you probably do a great deal of sitting every day—crouching over a desk, a computer, or a steering wheel. You will want to focus on formulating your yoga practice to address the muscular imbalances created by these activities.

Attempt to fully utilize yogic discipline in this process of balancing your body: be patient. Once you discover the specifics of your body and know where you are tight and what you want to strengthen, know and work graciously on accepting the fact that your body will not change overnight. It is important in yoga practice to accept where you're at at any given time. Yoga teaches us to face the circumstances of our current existence with faith, courage, nobility, and calm. Walk gently amid the obstacles that seem to stand in the way of where you think you ought to be. Work with your body, not against it, and have patience with your process and the lessons inherent therein. It is these very lessons that spin the rich fabric of our lives. Having patience with our process and the circumstances in which we find ourselves gives us the opportunity to touch into the energy that helps us to forge the traits that assist us in approaching life with courage and nobility, as well as with the steadiness (sthira) and comfort (sukha) of the peaceful yogic warrior.

Go forth. Walk gently on your path.

# 6

# Body Balance,
# Mind Balance

As children we engaged in lots of activities that trained our balancing skills. Remember playing hopscotch, or skipping on one leg, or playing tug-of-war? We didn't think of these activities as balance training—we just did them naturally.

Balance—the marvelous ability to regain equilibrium when the body is taken off center—can be regarded as our sixth sense. When balance is good a person is able to recover equilibrium in a timely fashion and is more often than not successful in doing so. This ability to maintain or regain steadiness is controlled by the vestibular system, which is housed in the inner ear. You may be able to remember a time when an inner ear infection affected your body's sense of balance. Even though it is a temporary condition the event is one that most people do not easily forget, since every step a person takes is affected by the vestibular system's ability to work properly.

Every time your body is required to perform its balancing function a complex sequence of events takes place. Sensory organs called proprioceptors, located in the skin, muscles, and joints, advise your brain about what your body's position is; your eyes retrieve environmental information and relay that to the brain as well. The nervous system then relays messages to your muscles based on this information that it gleans from the equilibrium centers in the brain. The muscles lengthen or contract in order to keep you balanced on your vertical axis.

Avid fitness enthusiasts and athletes must have a well-developed sense of balance to be effective in performing their sports. Think of the demands a hockey player places on his vestibular system. The hockey player's balance is constantly challenged as he monitors and maneuvers the puck and checks other players who are attempting to thwart his efforts. Similarly, the mountain biker's vestibular system must respond quickly to rocks, roots, and uneven surfaces on the paths and hillsides on which she rides. The challenge to a mountain bikers' balancing skills are constant and relentless. Cross-country runners are challenged in the same way.

It matters little what the sport is. In order to be proficient at his or her sport the athlete needs to be able to change the body's center of gravity to match the movements integral to the activity. Balance training helps to streamline movement by stimulating the nervous system to respond quickly to equilibrium challenges, discouraging unnecessary movement that causes the limbs to flail and generally waste precious energy.

Balance training is important for everybody. Most of us are unaware of the many controls that our bodies perform for us over the course of a day's activities. Stepping down from a curb or over something that lands in our path by surprise are activities where our body performs its unique balancing act, often without even a passing conscious thought from us.

By the time we are in our senior years our balancing skills decrease significantly unless we are involved in activities that help us to keep those skills well honed. Falls are a major cause of injury for the elderly—more than half of the accident-related deaths in the elderly population can be accounted for by falls. Well-designed balance-training programs help facilitate body awareness and stimulate the body's reflexes, both of which enhance confidence and improve quality of movement and thereby reduce the possibility of injury. One study reports that the tendency to fall can be reduced by 50 percent in healthy individuals as old as ninety when the body's reflexes are stimulated on a regular basis.

Balance training is also an integral component in rehabilitation, especially for those who have suffered musculoskeletal or nervous system injuries or stroke. The first step toward rehabilitation involves reeducating the body about proper alignment and neutral posture for the joint(s) involved. Initial efforts in rehabilitating an injury are therefore directed toward retraining the proprioception necessary to sense a joint's neutrality. Without appropriate balance training as part of one's rehabilitation reflexes and muscles do not work as quickly in detecting and responding to environmental conditions that can cause reinjury.

The activities we use to improve balance as adults mimic the games we played as children. Using the ball as a tool for this training takes balance development to a whole new level. When we practice balancing postures on a mat on the floor we can count on the floor's innate steadiness—the floor does not move. But when we use an exercise ball to practice balancing asanas we are provided with a greater challenge. The unsteady surface of the ball forces our stabilizing musculature, our proprioceptive organs, and our minds to function at optimal ability in order to successfully execute the asana.

Many of the postures presented in this chapter are classic yoga balance asanas adapted to use on the ball. Others are not balancing postures at all, yet the dynamic qualities of the ball let us modify the asana so that it becomes a balance challenge.

When the yogis designed balancing postures they were not meant to develop physical balance alone. Balancing postures provided yogis with a physical strategy that could help bring about mental stillness. By focusing their energies and slowing the breath they could hold the balancing postures for extended periods of time. The simple act of funneling the energy to focus the mind on a balancing posture helps to center the practitioner.

We all have those times when we feel like the world is spinning out of control around us and we are looking for an anchor—something to keep us from spinning too. You will most likely find that losing yourself in the act of holding a balancing posture helps to cultivate stillness and calm in a mind that was previously screaming with chatter. The yogic goal of the balancing postures is to promote balance and harmony within your entire being, balancing opposing energies along with the right and left sides of the body, binding your being together into a more fully integrated whole.

Balancing postures hone our concentration, focus, and discipline—these are the qualities required to enter and exit and, most important, to "hold" the posture. When working with the asanas in this chapter it is helpful to follow a few important principles to get the most out of your practice.

1. Before moving into any posture consciously slow the breath.
2. Slowly ease into the posture.
3. Find your dristi, a point of focus for your vision, which will help you in maintaining proper positioning of the asana as you breathe.
4. Notice the place where your feet are connecting with the ground. Focus on that place of solid contact. Spread the feet and toes so you have a solid base of contact. Breathe into the place where your feet are connecting with the earth.

5. If you feel that you are losing your balance, focus on slowing the breath even more to calm the mind. Draw in your transverse abdominis muscles and then attempt to release the pose rather than "falling" out of it.
6. Reposition yourself, slow your breath, and attempt the pose once again.
7. If you are shaking or swaying in the pose do not be concerned. Before slamming both feet down and giving up on the pose, engage the transverse abdominis and see if you can, in fact, hold the pose for a little longer, even if only for a few seconds.

The postures in this chapter are sequenced in order of difficulty so that you can progress slowly and systematically in strengthening your balancing skills. You may wish to choose two or three balancing postures to work on for several weeks; when you feel you have mastered one then substitute a new posture that increases the challenge. If you are using the posture to help you relax and center yourself, hold the posture for as long as feels comfortable to you. Once you feel grounded and centered in the posture drink in the sensation of being totally quiet, calm, still. At times it can feel almost as if you are floating. You probably will find you want to hold the posture for somewhere around thirty seconds. When you are ready to come out of the posture gently engage the transverse abdominis muscles, release the pose, and move on to another.

When practicing a posture as part of your fitness routine to improve your physical balancing skills, hold the posture for roughly ten seconds and then move on to another posture, progressing through a series of three or four balancing asanas at a fairly lively pace. Athletes may find it useful to settle into the posture and then begin to move an arm or a leg—a limb that is not involved in stabilizing the body at that moment—making a movement such as a small circle with the limb in order to create more of a balance challenge in the posture.

Regardless of your intention, read and understand the directions before you move into the posture so that once you are balancing you do not have to move out of the position to read or to look at images.

## The Asanas

## *Knee Lift*

The Knee Lift is an introductory balance exercise that will help to warm up your nervous system, including your brain, in preparation for the more advanced exercises to follow. The virtue of beginning your balance training with a fundamental exercise such as a knee lift is that it allows you to concentrate on one group of skills at a time. In performing a familiar movement, such as lifting the knee, you do not need to focus on learning the skills necessary to perform a new pose; you can devote the majority of your attention to fine-tuning the skills needed to stay upright.

**Purpose** To train balancing skills and to help the student feel more grounded and centered.

**Watchpoint** • Maintain a lengthened spine throughout the pose.

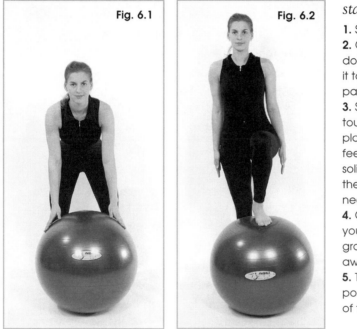

Fig. 6.1　Fig. 6.2

*starting position*

**1.** Stand facing your ball (fig. 6.1).
**2.** Observe what your breath is doing and then consciously change it to a slow diaphragmatic-breathing pattern.
**3.** Sense the place where your feet touch the ground. Focus on that place of solid contact. Spread the feet and toes so that you have a solid base of contact. Breathe into the place where your feet are connecting with the ground.
**4.** Continue to breathe calmly until you feel centered and strongly grounded in present-moment awareness.
**5.** These guidelines for the starting position are applicable to every one of the balancing poses.

*movement*

**1.** Continuing with your diaphragmatic breathing, build the following into your breath pattern when you are ready. Exhale and engage the transverse abdominis.
**2.** Lift your knee and place your foot on the ball without reverting to shallow breathing or holding the breath (fig. 6.2).
**3.** Find a dristi, a point of focus, on the wall and maintain your focus there with a soft gaze. Allow yourself to work from within, giving your attention only to the sensations within your body—focus on your breathing patterns and your sense of how steady you are. Sense how your confidence level regarding your ability to hold the pose and not fall out of it might be affecting your execution. Trust yourself.
**4.** Breathe in a rhythmic, diaphragmatic fashion. Maintain the position for three full breaths or until you cannot hold the posture without generating excess tension.
**5.** Release to the starting position.
**6.** Repeat on the other side.

# Tree Pose (Vrikshasana)

Tree pose is a basic level balancing pose. The essence of this pose communicates a number of positive images: trees grow tall toward the heavens but their roots are firmly planted within Mother Earth; trees weather many storms and maintain balance throughout the course of most. This posture stretches the inner thigh and the latissimus dorsi and improves core stability. Tree asana reminds us that, though the winds of change and adversity may blow, we can remain firmly and confidently rooted.

**Purpose** To train balancing skills and to help the practitioner feel grounded and centered. To improve core stability and strengthen the quadriceps. To stretch the latissimus dorsi and inner thigh.

**Watchpoints** • Maintain a lengthened spine throughout the pose. • Retract the chin to maintain neutral alignment through the cervical spine. • Balance your weight evenly on the standing foot. • Do not hold your breath.

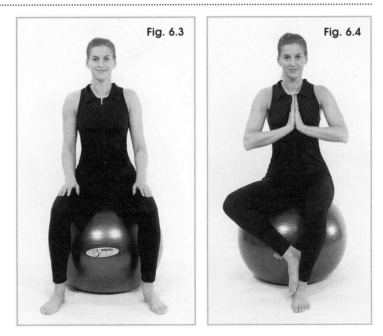

Fig. 6.3    Fig. 6.4

### starting position

**1.** Sit on the ball with feet shoulder-distance apart (fig. 6.3). Breathe in a slow, rhythmic, diaphragmatic manner.
**2.** Sense the place where your feet touch the ground. Focus on that place of solid contact. Spread the feet and toes so that you have a solid base of contact. Breathe into the place where your feet are connecting with the ground.
**3.** Continue to breathe calmly until you feel centered and strongly grounded in present-moment awareness.

### movement—level one

**1.** Maintain diaphragmatic breathing. On an exhale engage the transverse abdominis and gently retract the chin. Place the hands at the breastbone in prayer position.
**2.** Place the sole of the right foot on the inner side of the left ankle (fig. 6.4). The left leg will be the strong stabilizing force in this pose.

**3.** Maintain this position for as long as you can without generating excess tension. Continue breathing slowly from the diaphragm.
**4.** Return the right foot to the starting position.
**5.** Repeat on the other side of the body.

97

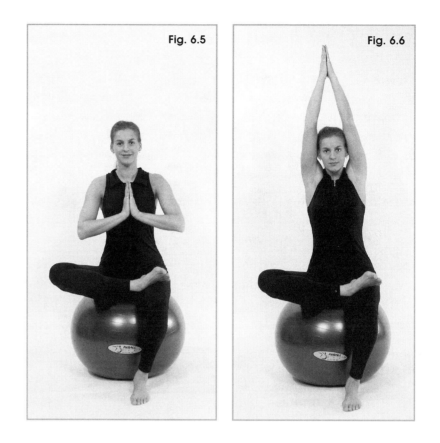

Fig. 6.5

Fig. 6.6

## movement—level two

**1.** Begin with the starting position setup described before "movement—level one."

**2.** Maintain diaphragmatic breathing. On an exhale engage the transverse abdominis and gently retract the chin. Place the hands at the breastbone in prayer position.

**3.** Place the right foot on top of the left thigh (fig. 6.5).

**4.** Maintain this position for as long as you can without generating excess tension. Continue breathing slowly from the diaphragm.

**5.** Return the right foot to the starting position.

**6.** Repeat on the other side of the body.

## movement—level three

**1.** Begin with the starting position setup described before "movement—level one."

**2.** Maintain diaphragmatic breathing. On an exhale engage the transverse abdominis and gently retract the chin. Place the hands at the breastbone in prayer position.

**3.** Place the right foot on top of the left thigh. Raise the arms overhead (fig. 6.6).

**4.** Maintain this position for as long as you can without generating excess tension. Continue breathing slowly from the diaphragm.

**5.** Return the right foot to the starting position.

**6.** Repeat on the other side of the body.

# Eagle Pose (Garudasana)

In Indian mythology the eagle is a deity and thus is considered sacred. This posture stretches the posterior shoulder muscles and the inner thigh. It strengthens the ankles, the quadriceps, and the gluteal muscles. The eagle represents prana, the life force. I believe the eagle reminds us all that we have unique talents and gifts that we bring to the world in order to fulfill our life's purpose here on Earth. In this way we live out the unique life force that the Great Spirit blessed us with from the vast heavens above.

**Purpose** To train balance skills and to help the student to feel centered. To strengthen the ankles, quadriceps, and gluteals. To stretch the posterior shoulder muscles and the inner thigh.

**Watchpoints** • Be sure that you don't twist your knee joint when wrapping one leg around the other. • Keep your spine long and aligned.

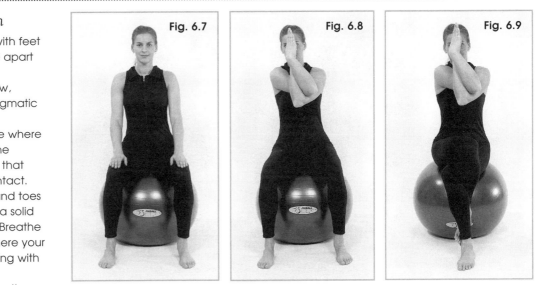

Fig. 6.7 Fig. 6.8 Fig. 6.9

*starting position*

**1.** Sit on the ball with feet shoulder-distance apart (fig. 6.7).
**2.** Breathe in a slow, rhythmic, diaphragmatic manner.
**3.** Sense the place where your feet touch the ground. Focus on that place of solid contact. Spread the feet and toes so that you have a solid base of contact. Breathe into the place where your feet are connecting with the ground.
**4.** Continue to breathe calmly until you feel centered and strongly grounded in present-moment awareness.

*movement*

**1.** Inhale and exhale. Engage the transverse abdominis.
**2.** Bend the elbows, lift the arms to chest height, and wrap the left arm over the right (fig. 6.8).
**3.** Lift the right leg and wrap it around the left leg (fig. 6.9).
**4.** Maintain this position for as long as you can without generating excess tension. Continue breathing slowly from the diaphragm.
**5.** Slowly return to the starting position.
**6.** Repeat on the other side of the body.

# Side Plank *(Vashishthasana)*

This asana is named after an Indian sage. Vashishthasana is a challenging pose. If you view this posture from the side it resembles a plank wedged between two panes of glass. In addition to fostering focus and determination this posture can help you in developing nonattachment to success or failure.

**Purpose** To train balancing skills and help the student feel centered. To strengthen the arms and shoulders. To improve core stability. To stretch the oblique abdominals and the intercostal muscles (the muscles between the ribs).

**Watchpoint** • Keep the hips "stacked," the upper hip in line with the lower.

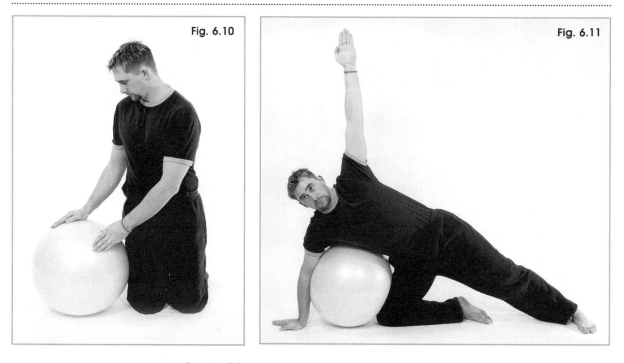

Fig. 6.10

Fig. 6.11

*starting position*

Kneel upright beside the ball. The ball is on your right side. Draw the ball close to the body (fig. 6.10).

*movement*

**1.** Drape your body over the side of the ball and stack the left hip on top of the right hip. The left leg is extended long, forming a straight line from heel to shoulder. Place the ball between the right arm and the bent right knee.

**2.** Reach the left arm to the ceiling (fig. 6.11).

**3.** Maintain this position for as long as you can without generating excess tension. Continue breathing slowly from the diaphragm.

**4.** Slowly return to the starting position.

**5.** Repeat on the other side of the body.

# Half Moon (Ardha Chandrasana)

This is an advanced balancing posture. This pose stretches and strengthens the oblique abdominals and the stabilizing musculature of the inner thigh while improving core stability and stretching the hamstrings. According to yogic theory the configuration of the body in Half Moon, trunk balanced over legs, looks like the moon placed in the sky. When executed correctly the arms should appear as if they are one long vertical line. Horizontally, there should be one long line from heel to head.

I find Half Moon to be a posture that develops grace and power. Grace develops with each attempt to move into the posture while keeping the body poised in one long line. The power center (core stability) improves as you challenge yourself to hold the pose for increasingly longer periods of time. Those with good balancing skills can challenge themselves further in Half Moon by moving the ball in small circles while trying to maintain balance.

**Purpose** To train balancing skills and help the student feel centered and grounded. To strengthen the oblique abdominals and the inner thigh. To improve core stability.

**Watchpoint** • Be careful not to twist the spine or arch the back while executing the pose.

*starting position*

**1.** Stand with the ball positioned on your right side. Turn your right foot toward the ball; the left foot points forward.
**2.** On the exhale engage the transverse abdominis.

*movement—level one*

**1.** Bend at the waist and place your right hand on the side of the ball; simultaneously raise your left leg off the floor approximately ten inches (fig. 6.12).
**2.** Attempt to hold this position for 6 seconds while you breathe rhythmically.
**3.** Inhale as you return to the starting position.
**4.** Repeat three to four times.
**5.** Repeat on the other side of the body.

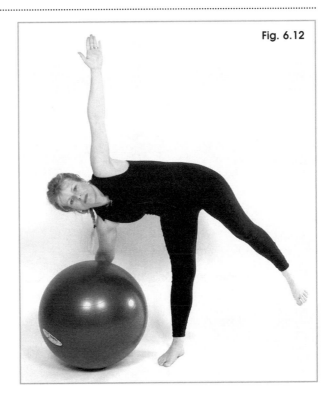

Fig. 6.12

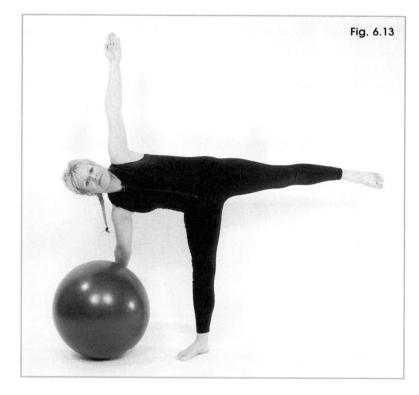

Fig. 6.13

*movement—level two*

**1.** Begin from the same starting position. Turn your right foot toward the ball; the left foot points forward.

**2.** On the exhale engage the transverse abdominis.

**3.** Exhale as you lift the left leg so that it is parallel with your hip. The body creates one long line from the heel to the top of the head (fig. 6.13).

**4.** Inhale as you return to the starting position.

**5.** Repeat three to four times.

**6.** Repeat on the other side of the body.

# Hand to Big Toe Posture
## (*Utthita hasta Padangusthasana*)

This asana is an advanced balancing posture. It is a challenge to maintain neutral spine while holding the toe. The challenge is increased further when the toe is brought out to the side. I feel that this posture fosters not only determination but risk taking.

**Purpose** To tone and strengthen the abdominals, to train balancing skills, to help the student feel grounded and centered.

**Watchpoint** • Be careful not to round the back as you lift the knee in the air.

*starting position*

Sit on the ball, feet parallel and shoulder-width apart (fig. 6.14).

*movement—level one*

**1.** Inhale. Exhale as you gently engage the transverse abdominis and anal sphincter muscles.

**2.** Lift your knee toward your chest until you can grasp the big toe on your right foot (fig. 6.15).

**3.** Straighten your leg as far as you are able to while still maintaining balance (fig. 6.16). Hold for 3 seconds.

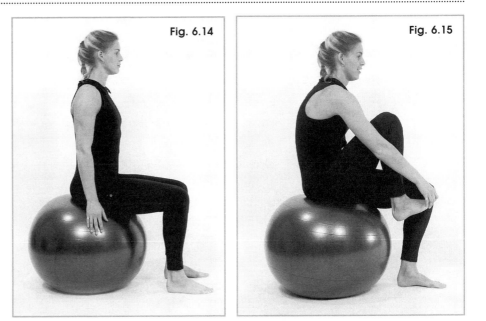

Fig. 6.14

Fig. 6.15

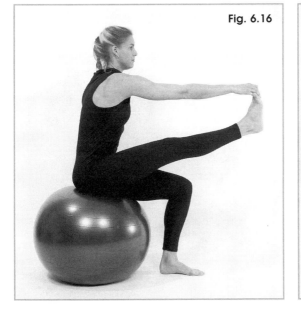

Fig. 6.16

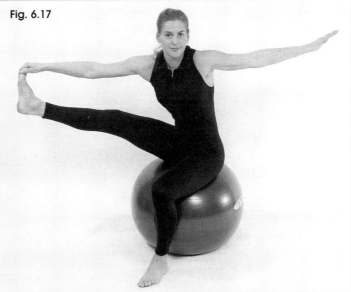

Fig. 6.17

**4.** Draw the leg out to the side and try to hold for 6 seconds (fig. 6.17).

**5.** Return to the starting position.

**6.** Repeat two to three times.

**7.** Repeat on the other side of the body.

# King Dancer (Natarajasana)

Nataraja is the name of the cosmic dancer, the Hindu god Siva. This asana is an advanced balancing posture. As you move into this elegant posture you may feel as if the dancer in you is eager to come alive.

**Purpose** To tone the muscles involved in stabilizing the core. To train balancing skills and help the student feel more grounded and centered. To stretch the quadriceps muscles.

**Watchpoint** • Be careful not to round the back as you lean forward.

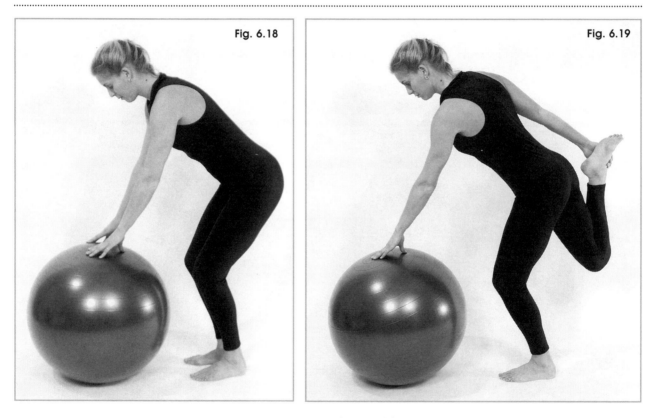

Fig. 6.18

Fig. 6.19

*starting position*

Stand facing your ball, knees bent and hands placed lightly on the top of the ball (fig. 6.18).

*movement—level one*

**1.** Bend your right knee, drawing your heel toward your buttocks. Grasp the foot with your right hand and hold (fig. 6.19). Your left knee is bent slightly. Your left hand is placed on the top surface of the ball.

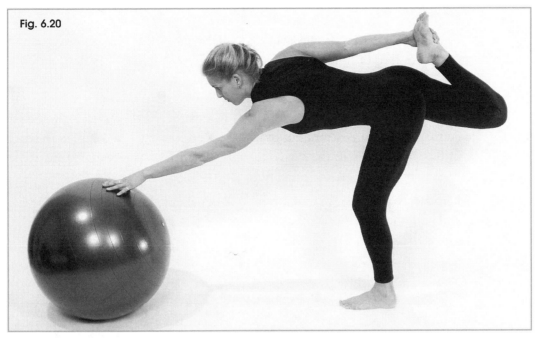

Fig. 6.20

**2.** Fold at the hip joint and slowly roll the ball forward as far as you are able (fig. 6.20). Keep the spine long—don't round the back or collapse through the chest in this position.

**3.** Attempt to hold this position for up to 10 seconds.

**4.** Return to the starting position.

**5.** Repeat on the other side.

### movement—level two

**1.** Bend your right knee, drawing your heel toward your buttocks. Grasp the foot with your right hand and hold. Your left knee is bent slightly. Your left hand is placed on the top surface of the ball.

**2.** Fold at the hip joint and slowly roll the ball forward until the upper body is approximately 45 degrees to the lower body. Keep the spine long.

**3.** Circle the ball first in a clockwise direction and then in a counterclockwise direction (fig. 6.21). This will considerably increase the balance challenge of this asana.

**4.** Repeat on the other side of the body.

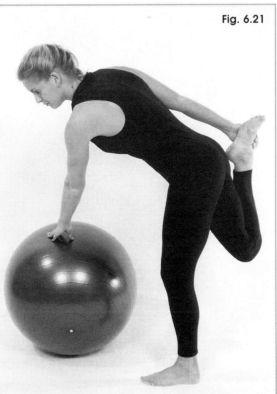

Fig. 6.21

# Candle Pose (Vaparita Karani Mudra)

Candle posture is so named because the shape of the body in this posture resembles that of a lit candle. Feel like the light on your candle is growing tired and burning out? Imagine it rekindling brightly as you practice this pose. This balancing posture differs from the others in that it is an inverted posture. This posture should never be practiced by people with cervical spine concerns. This posture reminds us that there is an internal fire going on in us all of the time known as the life force. The life force is sacred, something to be revered and thankful for.

**Purpose** To tone and strengthen the abdominal muscles, train balancing skills, and help the practitioner feel grounded and centered.

**Watchpoint** • If you have a neck injury avoid this posture. Remember that weight is to be centered over the chest, not over the head and neck.

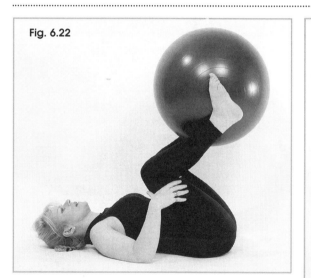

Fig. 6.22

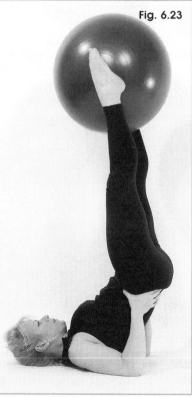

Fig. 6.23

## starting position

Lie on your back with your knees bent and the soles of the feet on the floor, the ball secured between the ankles.

## movement

**1.** On the exhale gently engage the transverse abdominis.
**2.** Exhale and slowly draw the knees toward the chest as you raise the ball from the ground (fig. 6.22).
**3.** Move your hands to your hip bones and let them support you as you inhale and gently lift your hips from the floor, raising them above your chest (fig. 6.23). Stop your upward lift of the hips at the point where you feel the chin "crunching" toward the chest. Align hips and elbows to ensure that there is no weight transferred to the neck.
**4.** Attempt to hold the posture here for up to 10 seconds.
**5.** Slowly lower the hips to the floor, using hands to support the hips in the down phase.

# Warrior 3 (Virabhadrasana 3)

This posture from the Warrior series is considered an advanced posture. I consider this progression from Warrior 1 and Warrior 2 to be the final preparation for true warriorship. In this posture the warrior develops perseverance and discipline through holding the pose. As you practice this posture envision your own sense of discipline and perseverance being fortified.

**Purpose** To tone and strengthen the abdominal muscles. To train balancing skills. To help the practitioner feel grounded and centered.

**Watchpoint** • Maintain a long spine throughout this posture.

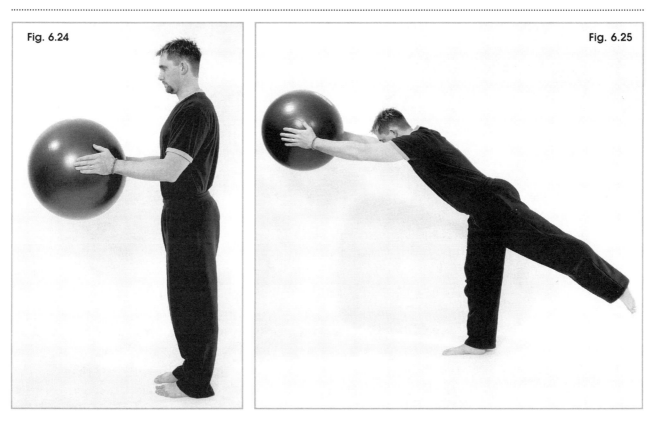

Fig. 6.24

Fig. 6.25

*starting position*

**1.** Stand with your feet shoulder-distance apart. Find neutral spine by using the Postural Setup.
**2.** Pick up the ball and hold it in front of your trunk (fig. 6.24).

*movement—level one*

**1.** Exhale and engage your transverse abdominis muscles.
**2.** Lean slightly forward and extend your arms as you press your left leg out behind you about eight inches (fig. 6.25). Hold this posture for 10 seconds, breathing rhythmically.

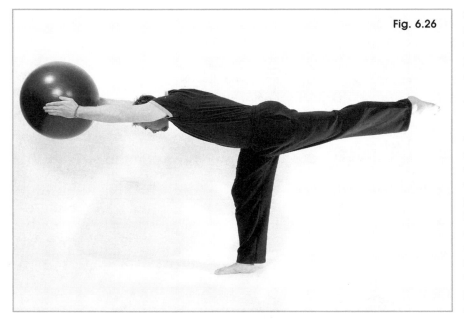

**Fig. 6.26**

**3.** Return to the starting position, Slowly and with control, release your arms toward the trunk as you place the extended leg on the floor.
**4.** Repeat on the other side.

*movement—level two*

**1.** From the same starting position as level one, extend your arms and raise the ball overhead as you flex at the hips and lean forward until the trunk and leg are parallel to the floor (fig. 6.26).
**2.** Attempt to hold this position for 6 seconds, breathing rhythmically.
**3.** Return to the starting position, Slowly and with control, release your arms toward the trunk as you place the extended leg on the floor.
**4.** Repeat on the other side.

Having adequate balance is a requirement for everyday living. Moving through the various balancing exercises helps us to systematically challenge our vestibular system and our core musculature so that we can hone our balancing skills. I suggest that you choose two to three balancing postures to perform every time you do your Yoga on the Ball practice. Select new postures every few weeks. This gives your body a new challenge and can sometimes provide the catalyst your body needs to mobilize your metabolism.

Remember that balancing exercises help to create equilibrium in your emotional and psychological life as well. The media saturation and fast pace of life in the twenty-first century gives us few opportunities for developing our powers of concentration; rather, our attention is split several different ways most of the time, and our brain waves move fast to keep up with the beta attention that is required in every waking moment.

Balancing postures help us to slow down. We are given the opportunity to shun multitasking and to focus on the present, on sensations and on breath. Smile into the moment. Breathe. Focus inward.

Integrate the balancing postures into your life as much as you can.

# 7

# The Advanced Postures

The asanas in this chapter are designed to meet the needs of the advanced exerciser. I recommend to people who want to attempt the challenging postures here that they already be well conditioned and have considerable experience working with both the exercise ball and hatha yoga postures. Combining yoga postures with the ball takes a yoga practice to a completely new level, one that can provide unique challenges to even the most seasoned exercisers and athletes.

People who wish to work with the asanas in this chapter quite likely have a predetermined goal relevant to their preferred sport or fitness activity. For instance, my friend Alex, who was fortunate enough to retire younger than most folks, spends many of his leisure hours windsurfing along the coastlines of the countries he travels. Practicing advanced yoga postures on the unstable surface of the ball replicates the conditions Alex experiences on his windsurfing board. This allows him to train for his favorite leisure-time activity without even entering the water.

For Teri, an aspiring professional figure skater, executing the advanced yoga ball postures helps condition her vestibular system as well as her muscles for most efficiently utilizing the momentum she generates in her jumps and spins.

Kathi's goal is completely different. She is continually on the lookout for new physical challenges that will help her maintain a positive mind-set. Three years ago Kathi's husband was killed in a tragic accident; Kathi began running marathons to help her cope with her grief. The advanced Yoga on the Ball postures presented in the book provide her with a satisfying ongoing challenge that she can work at during any season of the year. Her well-conditioned body needs novel training opportunities to support her goals with respect to running marathons, and her determined spirit needs to be fed.

The various training needs of these individuals can be accomplished with regular practice of the asanas presented in this chapter. Consider your own training needs. Is there a particular sport you want to excel at? Are you trying to find your competetive edge, or is your desire to develop a training program that can support a lifestyle choice?

The advanced Yoga on the Ball postures can be the ultimate training tool. Athletes who rely solely on machine training suffer from a disadvantage because they do not reap the benefits of the increased nervous system activation brought about by the Yoga on the Ball advanced asana training. Also, because machines have stable contact with the floor the athlete does not get the experience of stabilizing his body on various planes—which is exactly what he needs to do in his playing environment. This allows his body to essentially practice many of the motor-recruitment patterns that will be demanded of him in performing his sport.

As in the earlier part of the workout outlined in the book, pay close attention to engaging the transverse abdominis as you work your way through the various asanas ahead. Engaging the transverse abdominis is particularily important to athletes as it helps the body to maintain its balance on the vertical axis. The moment an athlete engages the transverse abdominis she is creating greater containment and compression in her body, which helps to generate more control and power with respect to movement.

Before you practice any of the asanas here be certain that you are stabilized in the starting position. Progress slowly. If you are unable to complete an exercise, note it in your journal and pursue it again when you feel you have greater stability, coordination, strength, or flexibility.

## The Asanas

## *Supine Straight Leg Spinal Twist*

This pose stretches the rotator muscles of the spine. This posture also challenges the core muscles to stabilize the trunk properly as the legs are incrementally lowered toward the floor.

The adductor muscles, the muscles of the inside thigh that move the leg toward or across the midline of the body, are also worked in this posture, as they must contract isometrically in order to grip the ball. I find this to be a very artistic pose to observe from the top of the body when the asana is executed properly, with the body aligned in ideal posture and the pose being performed with precision and control. It is beautiful to see the angles of the leg relative to the trunk and the work the core musculature must do to stabilize the body as the legs lower to the floor.

**Purpose** To stretch the spinal rotator muscles and the muscles of the inner thigh. To stretch the muscles of the outer thigh.

**Watchpoints** • Maintain scapular stabilization throughout the asana. • Ensure that you actively control the lowering of the legs with the activation of the transverse abdominis so that there is no torque put on the spine that could leave it vulnerable to injury. • Be sure to move slowly and with control.

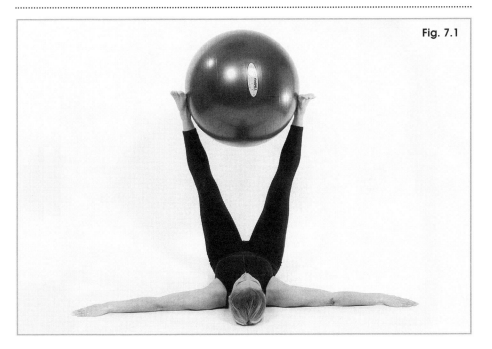

**Fig. 7.1**

*starting position*

**1.** Lie on your back on the floor. Extend the arms long from the shoulder girdle and engage the rhomboid muscles to retract the shoulder blades. The ball is positioned between the ankles.
**2.** Exhale and engage the transverse abdominis, then lift the legs to form a 90-degree angle to the trunk (fig. 7.1).
**3.** Inhale.

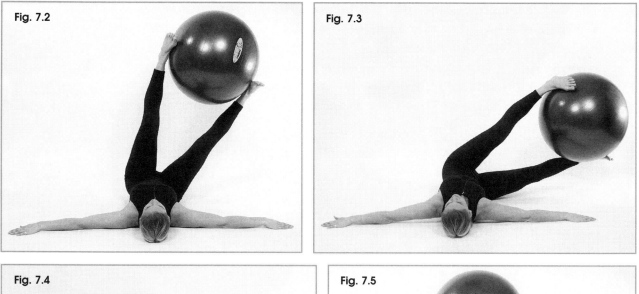

Fig. 7.2

Fig. 7.3

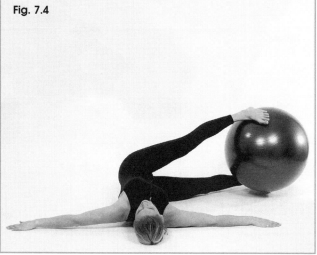

Fig. 7.4

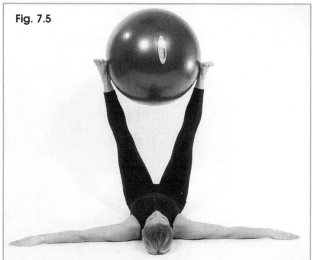

Fig. 7.5

*movement*

1. On the exhale, engage the transverse abdominis as you slowly lower your legs to the right, maintaining the 90-degree angle of the legs and trunk. Your eventual destination is the floor, but you want to take three moves to get there (figs. 7.2, 7.3, and 7.4). Control the lowering of the legs with an active transverse abdominis so you do not torque the spine. Attempt to hold each incremental change for 3 seconds.

2. Once the legs are at the floor, inhale, exhale, and inhale, maintaining a strong transverse abdominis activation.

3. Exhale as you lift the legs to return to the start position (fig. 7.5).

4. Repeat on the other side.

## *Yoga Chair Pose with Squat*

This is an advanced version of the Chair Pose—lifting one leg off the ground and placing it on the ball adds challenge to the traditional Chair pose. As you press the buttocks out behind you pretend that you are sitting back into a chair. When I practice this posture I am struck by the amount of control it takes to hold this posture once I have lowered myself into the "down" phase.

**Purpose** To improve core stability and tone the abdominal muscles. To tone the quadriceps, the gluteals, and the hamstrings. To stretch the latissimus dorsi.

**Watchpoints** • Make sure the knee is lined up over the ankle and does not press out over the toe. • Maintain scapular stabilization throughout the asana.

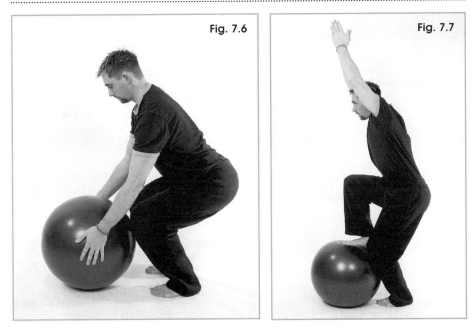

Fig. 7.6

Fig. 7.7

*starting position*

**1.** Stand with your feet slightly wider than hip-distance apart, the ball on the ground in front of you. Engage the rhomboid muscles to draw the shoulder blades toward the spine and stabilize the scapulae.

**2.** Squat down and take hold of the ball (fig. 7.6). Press your buttocks out behind you as if you were going to sit in a chair. Maintain an elongated spine and scapular retraction.

*movement*

**1.** Exhale and engage the transverse abdominis, then raise the arms overhead and place one foot on the ball (fig. 7.7). Continue to press the buttocks out behind you. Pause for 3 seconds, breathing and maintaining a strong transverse abdominis.

**2.** Return to the starting position.

**3.** Repeat on the other side.

**4.** Repeat up to eight times on each side.

## Balancing Yogi

Balancing Yogi is a challenging exercise. Your skill will improve rapidly with practice once you sense how to situate your body and use your core musculature to balance properly. Those who engage in sports such as windsurfing, skateboarding, or roller blading will find this posture useful because it coaxes the body to replicate the same movements necessary to maintain balance in those sports. Balancing Yogi is almost certain to bring out the playful side of you. If I have had a particularily stressful day I begin my workout with this posture as it never fails to help me crack a smile. And once my brain changes from the experience of that first smile the rest of my workout is much more manageable and pleasurable.

**Purpose** To train balancing skills. To tone and strengthen the abdominal muscles and improve core stability.

**Watchpoints** • Keep the spine lengthened and in neutral position. • Maintain scapular stabilization throughout the asana.

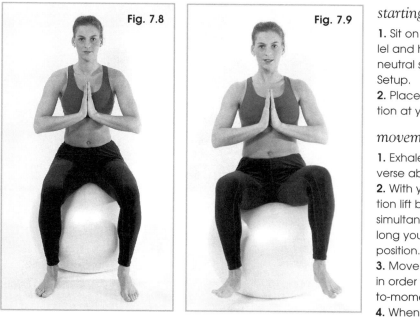

Fig. 7.8

Fig. 7.9

*starting position*

**1.** Sit on the ball with the feet parallel and hip-distance apart. Find neutral spine by using the Postural Setup.
**2.** Place your hands in prayer position at your breastbone (fig. 7.8).

*movement*

**1.** Exhale and engage the transverse abdominis.
**2.** With your hands in prayer position lift both feet off the ground simultaneously (fig. 7.9). See how long you can balance in this position.
**3.** Move your arms as you need to in order to fine-tune your moment-to-moment balancing skills.
**4.** When you wish to exit from this posture simply allow the weight of your body to pull you forward so that your feet touch the ground.

# Yoga Plank with Arm Work

In this asana you work to maintain balance while moving your arms as if they were the hands of a clock moving through time in that predictable circular motion. This is an effective balancing exercise—move slowly with impeccable control. Make sure you do not begin to droop at the midriff after a shift in your clock motion. This is a useful exercise for self-care of the back if you have back problems that are a result of instability in the spine.

**Purpose** To improve core stability. To tone the abdominals, arms, chest, and shoulders.

**Watchpoints** • Maintain a straight and elongated spine through this asana. • Breathe smoothly and calmly throughout the exercise. • Maintain scapular stabilization.

*starting position*

**1.** Stand with your feet shoulder-distance apart, the ball on the ground in front of you. Initiate scapular stabilization.
**2.** Come down to a kneeling position on the floor, your hands resting on either side of the ball (fig. 7.10).
**3.** Lay over the ball and walk out until the ball rests at the upper thighs (fig. 7.11). The hands are directly below the shoulder joints.
**4.** Engage the buttocks and squeeze the thighs together so that the sides of the knees are lightly touching each other. Imagine that your body is pointing at the 12-o'clock position (fig. 7.12).

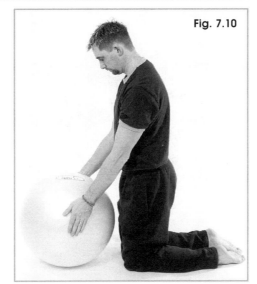

Fig. 7.10

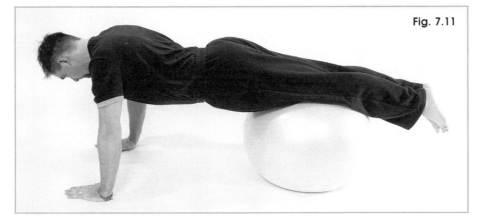

Fig. 7.11

115

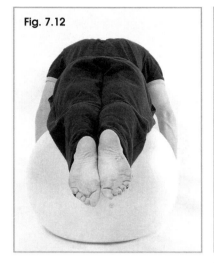

Fig. 7.12

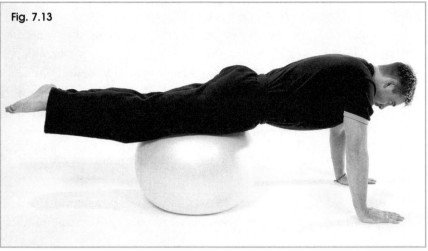

Fig. 7.13

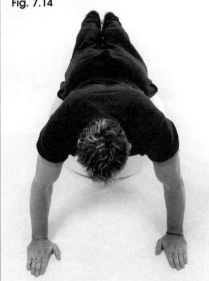

Fig. 7.14

## movement

**1.** On the exhale engage the transverse abdominis. Begin slowly "walking" your hands to the right. Allow your ball and your body to move with you as you travel.

**2.** Continue traveling until you complete one-quarter of the circle; stop at 3 o'clock and hold for 6 seconds (fig. 7.13).

**3.** Rest if you need to and then walk another quarter circle to 6 o'clock (fig. 7.14). Hold for 6 seconds.

**4.** Proceed to the next quarter hour when you are ready (fig. 7.15).

**5.** Continue on to the 12 o'clock position.

**6.** Rest here and then continue in the other direction when you are ready.

**7.** Perform one rotation in each direction.

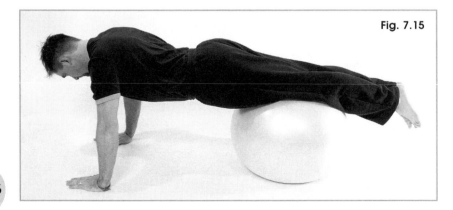

Fig. 7.15

# Yoga Plank with Push-Ups

This is another advanced variation of Plank pose. It is extremely challenging to keep yourself steady on the ball while executing push-ups. This posture requires upper body strength and a great deal of core stability to be able to maintain steadiness on the ball. The body should remain in one long line throughout the exercise, and shoulders should remain down and relaxed at all times.

This is an excellent exercise for wind surfers as it not only strengthens the muscles responsible for holding the sail in place but also strengthens the core musculature responsible for keeping the surfer in the upright position.

This asana is also useful for bodybuilders. Bodybuilders are known for their pectoral strength but often lack in the ability to stabilize the body to sustain holding heavy loads.

**Purpose** To tone and strengthen the abdominals, arms, chest and shoulders. To improve core stability.

**Watchpoints** • Maintain a straight spine throughout the posture. Do not arch the back. • Maintain scapular stabilization.

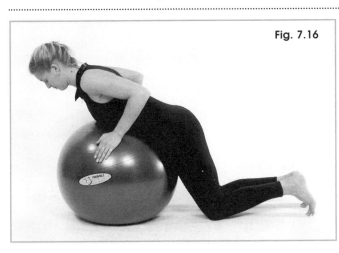

Fig. 7.16

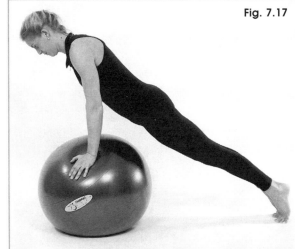

Fig. 7.17

*starting position*

**1.** Stand with your feet shoulder-distance apart, the ball on the ground in front of you. Engage the rhomboid muscles to draw the shoulder blades toward the spine and stabilize the scapulae.
**2.** Come down to a kneeling position on the floor, your hands resting on either side of the ball.
**3.** Lay over the ball and walk out until your chest is centered over the ball (fig. 7.16).

*movement*

**1.** Exhale and engage the transverse abdominis.
**2.** Inhale and lift your body up off the ball by straightening the arms (fig. 7.17). Maintain a strong lift through the spine and transverse abdominal engagement to keep you steady on the ball.
**3.** Exhale as you lower your body to the starting position.
**4.** Repeat this movement up to eight times.

## Advanced Prayer Roll Out

The next three asanas require the body to maintain stabilization as movement is introduced. These asanas are useful for training core musculature.

Prayer Roll Out will challenge those who have superb balancing skills and a strong upper body. The most common training error with this asana is arching the back as you roll out into the pose or losing transverse abdominis activation while executing the posture. Be certain that you have mastered the basic version of Prayer Roll Out before attempting this asana.

**Purpose** To improve core stability. To strengthen the abdominal muscles.

**Watchpoints** • Do not arch your back when rolling into this posture. • Maintain scapular stabilization throughout the asana. • Avoid this exercise if you have shoulder or rotator cuff problems.

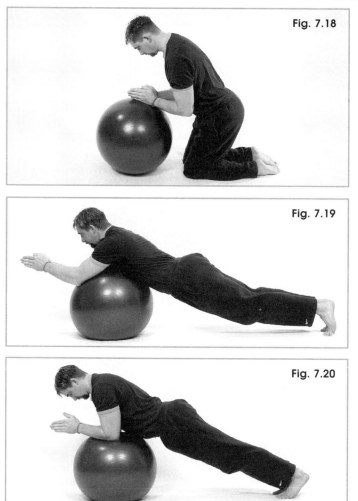

Fig. 7.18

Fig. 7.19

Fig. 7.20

*starting position*

**1.** Stand with your feet shoulder-distance apart, the ball on the ground in front of you. Engage the rhomboid muscles to draw the shoulder blades toward the spine and stabilize the scapulae.
**2.** Come down to a kneeling position in front of the ball. Bend your elbows and place your hands and wrists on the ball, palms facing inward in prayer position (fig. 7.18).

*movement*

**1.** Exhale and engage the transverse abdominis.
**2.** Keeping your hands in place on the ball, inhale as you lift the hips and extend the legs behind you, rolling the ball away from the body (fig. 7.19). The ball will be under the upper arms. Think of creating a straight, strong line from the heels to the fingertips.
**3.** Exhale as you roll the ball back in toward the body, maintaining neutral spine (fig. 7.20).
**4.** Repeat up to eight times.

# Advanced Bridge with Roll Out

In this advanced version of the Bridge asana you will need to focus your present-moment awareness on moving slowly and with control. Most students find it a challenge to remember to breathe while executing this exercise.

**Purpose** To tone and strengthen the abdominals and hamstrings. To improve core stability.

**Watchpoints** • Make sure you don't arch the back or lift your hips too high in the air. The idea is to make a straight line with the shoulders, hips, and knees.
• Be sure the neck is relaxed and the shoulders are drawn away from the ears.
• Maintain scapular stabilization throughout the asana.

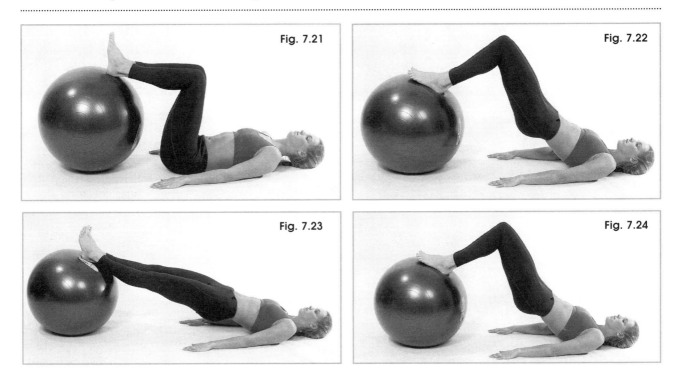

Fig. 7.21

Fig. 7.22

Fig. 7.23

Fig. 7.24

*starting position*

**1.** Lie on your back with your knees bent, heels resting on the ball and arms resting by the side of your thighs (fig. 7.21).
**2.** Engage the rhomboid muscles to draw the shoulder blades toward the spine and stabilize the scapulae.

*movement*

**1.** Exhale and engage the transverse abdominis.
**2.** Lift your hips from the floor so that your buttocks line up with the heels (fig. 7.22).
**3.** Inhale and extend the legs to roll the ball away from the body (fig. 7.23). Hold for 3 seconds.

**4.** Exhale as you roll the ball back in toward the body, maintaining the lift through the buttocks and hips (fig. 7.24).
**5.** Inhale and exhale here. On the exhale engage the transverse abdominis.
**6.** Repeat the asana up to eight times.

119

# Advanced Bridge with Roll Out and Leg Raise

In this exercise your balance is challenged even more than in the previous asana because you have the support of one leg only. When practicing this posture be certain that you do not sacrifice your form. It is essential that you maintain neutral spine and pelvis throughout the entire execution of this posture. If you feel yourself struggling excessively you need to breathe in a more relaxed fashion. If this does not help, work at the previous posture until you improve your strength and stability.

**Purpose** To tone and strengthen the abdominals. To improve core stability.

**Watchpoints** • Don't arch the back or lift the hips too high in this asana. The idea is to make a straight line with the shoulders, hips, and knees. Don't let the buttocks drop toward the floor. • Relax the neck and draw the shoulders away from the ears. • Maintain scapular stabilization throughout the asana. • If you are not able to use the breath rhythm as it is described just simply breathe smoothly and calmly without holding your breath.

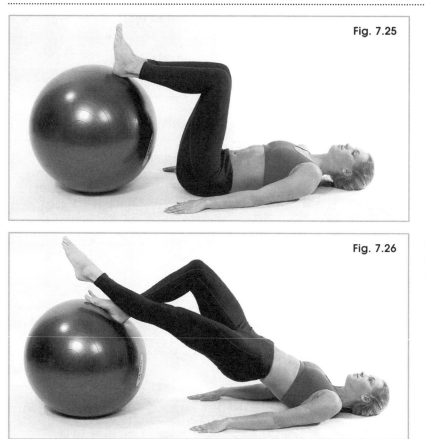

Fig. 7.25

Fig. 7.26

*starting position*

**1.** Lie on your back with your knees bent, heels resting on the ball and arms resting by the side of your thighs (fig. 7.25). **2.** Engage the rhomboid muscles to draw the shoulder blades toward the spine and stabilize the scapulae.

*movement*

**1.** Exhale and engage the transverse abdominis, then lift the hips from the floor. Extend the left leg and extend the right ankle to rest the right foot on the ball (fig. 7.26). Keep the ball in position.

**2.** Inhale and straighten the right leg to roll the ball away from the body (fig. 7.27).
**3.** Hold this position for up to 3 seconds.
**4.** Exhale and, using the right leg only, roll the ball back in toward the body. Lower the buttocks to the floor. Knees are bent and aligned over the hips. Both heels rest on the ball (fig. 7.28).
**5.** Repeat on the other side.

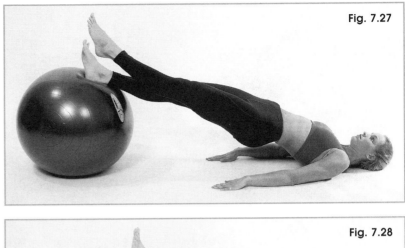

Fig. 7.27

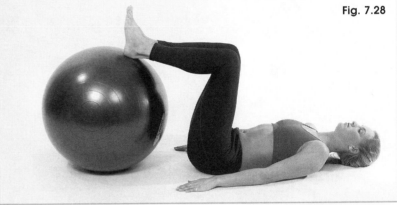

Fig. 7.28

## Side-Lying Plank

This variation of Plank pose gives you an option for strengthening the hip abductors, the muscles that move the leg away from the body's midline. The abductors include the gluteus muscles, the tensor fasciae latae, sartorius, and the deep muscles of the hip. You will need to experiment to find out which level of this exercise is appropriate for you. Use your balancing skills to maintain a long, lean line throughout the duration of the yoga exercise.

**Purpose** To strengthen the hip abductors. To improve core stability.

**Watchpoints** • Keep the top hip stacked over the bottom hip. • Don't twist or sidebend the spine. • Maintain scapular stabilization throughout the asana.

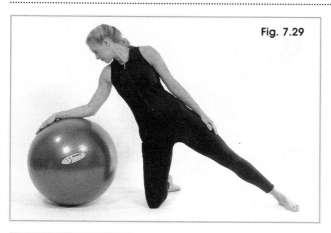

Fig. 7.29

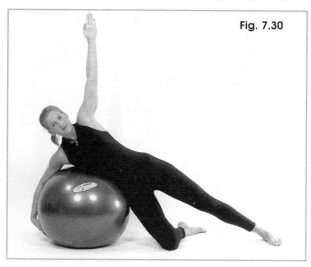

Fig. 7.30

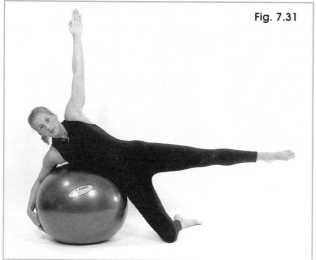

Fig. 7.31

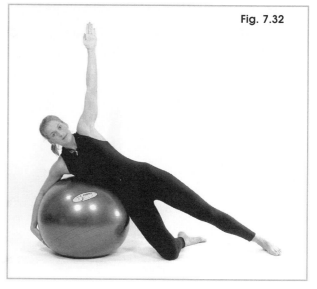

Fig. 7.32

## starting position

**1.** Kneel upright with your ball to the right of you. Engage the rhomboid muscles to draw the shoulder blades toward the spine and stabilize the scapulae.

**2.** Exhale and engage the transverse abdominis. Maintaining the spine in a straight line, lean toward the ball as you extend your left leg to the side (fig. 7.29). Inhale.

**3.** Exhale and drape the right side of your body over the ball, stacking the top hip over the bottom hip. Raise the left arm so that it is directly in line with the shoulder joint (fig. 7.30). Inhale.

## movement—level one

**1.** On the exhale engage the transverse abdominis.

**2.** Inhale. Exhale and engage the gluteal and thigh muscles to lift the top leg (fig. 7.31). Hold for 3 seconds.

**3.** Exhale as you release the top leg (fig. 7.32).

**4.** Repeat on the other side.

## movement—level two

**1.** Kneel upright with your ball to the right of you. Engage the rhomboid muscles to draw the shoulder blades toward the spine and stabilize the scapulae.

**2.** Exhale and engage the transverse abdominis. Maintaining the spine in a straight line, lean toward the ball as you extend both legs out to the side, stacking the hips and ankles. Extend the left arm above your head

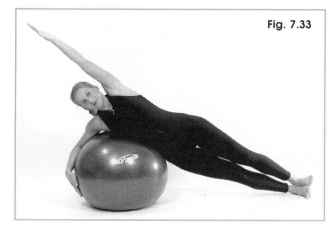

Fig. 7.33

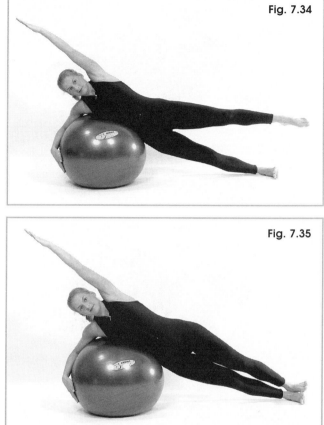

Fig. 7.34

Fig. 7.35

at a diagonal; feel a long, straight line from ankle to hip to fingertips (fig. 7.33).

**3.** Inhale and raise the top leg so that it is parallel with the floor (fig. 7.34). Hold for 3 seconds.

**4.** Exhale and release the leg to starting position (fig. 7.35).

**5.** Repeat on the other side.

## Side-Lying Plank with Twist

This advanced version of Side Plank is a challenging balance posture. It is difficult to simply hold the Side Plank, let alone keep control when you add movement to the equation. It is important to move through this asana slowly—maintaining a diaphragmatic breathing pattern makes it easier to achieve proper positioning. Be careful not to hold your breath as you work with this exercise.

**Purpose** To improve core stability. To tone the abdominal muscles. To strengthen the muscles of the arms and shoulders.

**Watchpoints** • Maintain the spine in a long, straight line. • Maintain scapular stabilization throughout the asana.

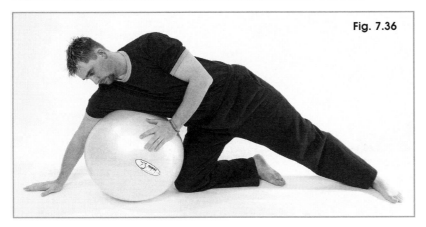

**Fig. 7.36**

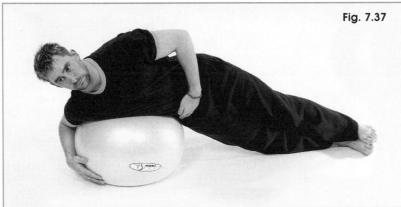

**Fig. 7.37**

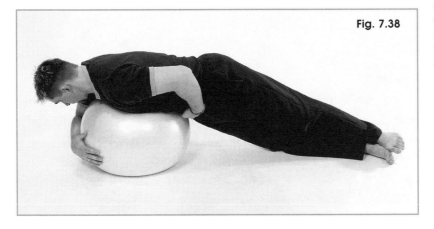

**Fig. 7.38**

*starting position*

Kneel upright with the ball to the right of you. Engage the rhomboid muscles to draw the shoulder blades toward the spine and stabilize the scapulae.

*movement*

**1.** Exhale and engage the transverse abdominis.

**2.** Lean to the right and drape your upper body over the ball so that the trunk rests securely on the ball. The right hand supports you on the floor, the left leg extends long (fig. 7.36). Inhale.

**3.** Exhale as you straighten the right leg and place the left hand on the belly (fig. 7.37). Make sure the hips are stacked.

**4.** Inhale and make a slight twist of your trunk toward the ball (fig. 7.38). This is a spinal rotation—make sure to maintain the spine's vertical axis as you rotate.

**5.** Hold this position for only a second.

**6.** Perform up to eight repetitions of this asana.

**7.** Repeat on the other side of the body.

# Advanced Down Dog

Be certain you have mastered the basic Down Dog (see page 64) before you progress to this advanced version. It is extremely challenging to work a posture when the body is inverted; breathe smoothly and calmly. This version of Down Dog tones the gluteals and strengthens the core and upper body.

**Purpose** To tone and strengthen the arms, shoulders, chest, and buttocks. To create space between the vertebrae by providing slight traction for the spine.

**Watchpoints** • Maintain a lengthened spine throughout this asana. • Keep the knees and shoulders slightly bent. • Maintain scapular stabilization. • Use relaxed yoga breathing throughout the asana.

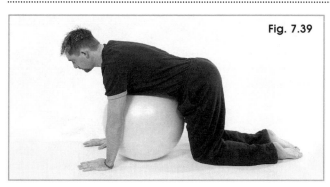

Fig. 7.39

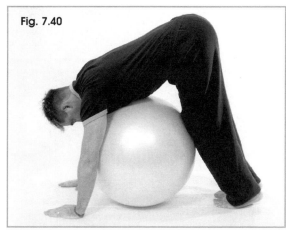

Fig. 7.40

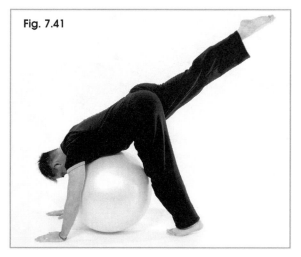

Fig. 7.41

## starting position

**1.** Stand with your feet slightly wider than hip-distance apart, the ball on the ground in front of you. Initiate scapular stabilization.
**2.** Kneel in front of the ball. Place your hands palms down on the floor. Walk out until the ball is supporting the chest and the wrists are directly under the shoulder joints (fig. 7.39).
**3.** Exhale and engage the transverse abdominis. Press into the hands as you flex the hips and lift the buttocks into the air. Your upper body and trunk will form an inverted V (fig. 7.40).

## movement

**1.** Exhale and engage the transverse abdominis.
**2.** Inhale. Exhale as you extend your right leg back, aligning the ankle with the shoulder joint (fig. 7.41).
**3.** Hold this leg extension for 3 seconds.
**4.** Return to the starting position.
**5.** Repeat for up to eight repetitions.
**6.** Repeat on the other side.

125

# Yoga Plank Hover

The following asanas are directed at the abdominals. These postures will help to develop an aeshetically pleasing look through the trunk and improve the stability of the spine.

Yoga Plank Hover is a variation of Plank pose. This exercise improves core stability and tones the abdominals. Record the length of time that you are able to hold this pose when you first try it, and then work to slowly increase the time you are able to maintain it. I recommend that you hold the posture for a minimum of 30 seconds and work up to holding it for 1 minute, but the first few times you practice the asana you may not get anywhere near this holding time.

**Purpose** To strengthen the spinal stabilizers. To tone the abdominal muscles.

**Watchpoints** • Work to create a straight line from head to toe. • Maintain scapular stabilization throughout the asana.

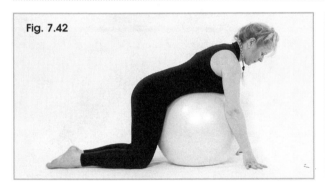

Fig. 7.42

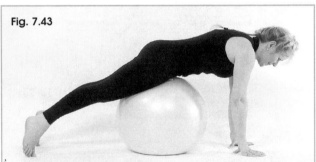

Fig. 7.43

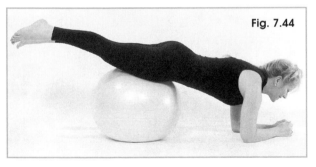

Fig. 7.44

*starting position*

**1.** Stand with your feet slightly wider than hip-distance apart, the ball on the ground in front of you. Initiate scapular syabilization.
**2.** Come to kneeling. Drape your trunk over the ball and roll forward into Cat position (fig. 7.42).

*movement—level one*

**1.** Exhale and engage the transverse abdominis. Slowly walk out on the ball until the ball is underneath the hips and upper thighs (fig. 7.43). Inhale.
**2.** Exhale as you bend the elbows and lift the legs from the floor to center your upper body weight on your forearms (fig. 7.44).
**3.** Attempt to hold the position for at least 30 seconds and up to 1 minute.

*movement—level two*

1. From the same starting position, slowly walk out on the ball until the ball is underneath the shins and ankles. Inhale.
2. Exhale as you bend the elbows and center your upper body weight on your forearms (fig. 7.45). Maintain strong transverse abdominis engagement.
3. Attempt to hold this position for at least 30 seconds and up to 1 minute.

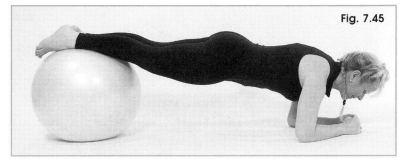

**Fig. 7.45**

# Rolling Tabletop

We finish our survey of advanced Yoga on the Ball postures with this intensive version of the Tabletop asana. This posture provides an extreme balance challenge; the key is to maintain transverse abdominis activation and neutral spine and pelvis throughout the asana. This asana promotes the development of coordination and agility. It is useful to those who take part in "extreme" sports, as it challenges the body to maintain control throughout an exercise that requires agility, coordination, and risk taking. The risk-taker who wants greater challenge can continue to incrementally increase speed as her skill improves.

**Purpose** To tone and strengthen the abdominal muscles. To improve core stability.

**Watchpoints** • Maintain an elongated, straight spine throughout the asana. • Keep the buttocks lifted. • Breathe smoothly and calmly throughout the asana.

*starting position*

1. Sit on the ball with the feet parallel and hip-distance apart. Find neutral spine by using the Postural Setup.
2. Walk your feet out and carefully let the ball roll under you until your head and neck are totally supported by the ball. Make sure your hips and buttocks are lifted.
3. Extend your arms out to your sides.

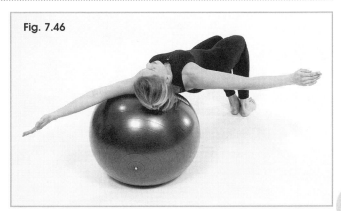

**Fig. 7.46**

127

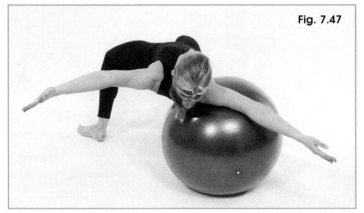

**Fig. 7.47**

*movement*

**1.** Exhale and engage the transverse abdominis. Keep the buttocks lifted as you begin to slowly walk your feet to the right (fig. 7.46). The ball will roll as you move.

**2.** When you reach your far right position, resituate yourself securely on the ball and then walk your feet back to the center.

**3.** Repeat on the other side (fig. 7.47).

**4.** Repeat two or three more times on each side.

Improvement in execution of the asanas in this chapter is all about refinement of the postures. Work diligently at using your muscles actively to create long, lean yoga lines for each and every posture. Each time you practice, attempt to sculpt even more distinct linear creations with your body. If you have the luxury of practicing in front of a mirror you will want to see strong angles and lines. Regardless of whether you are training for sport or leisure activity, for physical conditioning or mental toughness, choose the postures that uniquely match the demands placed on your body and mind. Refrain from overpracticing the poses at which you excel in order to prevent muscle imbalance and overtraining of specific muscle groups.

# 8
# Relaxation and Restoration

Walking along the wooded path by the river behind my home with my silver-haired Siberian husky restores me deeply. I can feel all the fragmented pieces of mind, body, and soul coming together. My breath begins to slow the minute my feet step onto the path. I close my eyes for a second, listening to the sounds of broken twigs and old leaves crackling under my feet. I fall into a soft tratak, a relaxed gaze, as I absorb into my soul the vibrant colors of the lush ever-greens surrounding me. From time to time I slowly swivel my head toward the river, sensing the flow of the water. My eyes catch sight of the wavelike ripples of the river's current and I lazily track the movement. I feel myself becoming almost mesmerized by the water's motion as the tensions of the day slowly slough away and seem to drift off down the river.

As I continue to walk along the path I feel a strong sense of communion . . . with Mother Earth, with the waterfowl and animals that inhabit the space around me, and with the vast intelligence that created it all. I offer up my gratitude . . . and my heart's desires. I receive peace. It permeates further into my body with each step that I take. I am home.

I relish the serenity of being in this wooded paradise. It is symbolic of the nurturing haven within me—a quiet, calm center, that soulful place that exists in each of us that is nourished by the wavelike rhythm of the breath and by prayer, meditation, and quiet contemplation.

It is imperative that we fill our lives with frequent opportunities to refill the well of this quiet, calm center. Yoga, meditation, and relaxation can help us to keep that well "topped off" so we do not need to over-rely on reserves in stressful times. Taking a few moments in the morning before work or at day's end to luxuriate in relaxed breathing and restorative stretches can significantly improve your wellness quotient. Regularly taking part in a restorative activity trains the body and the mind to be able to reproduce the sensation of being relaxed when it's most needed: it's beneficial to be able to relax at will before you step into an important business meeting, have a tooth extracted at the dentist's office, or lay down for a night of replenishing sleep.

We know that restorative activities alter the brain's chemistry, upping levels of seretonin and other chemicals that help us to feel more optimistic and energetic and less uptight. These chemicals take effect at the cellular level—studies show that people who are generally more positive are typically healthier. Conversely, people who exhibit traits such as impatience or negativity tend to be sick more often and have increased incidence of high blood pressure. Furthermore, people who experience a catastrophic event such as losing a loved one will often fall prey to serious illness in the year or so following the loss or tragedy. It is exceedingly important to pay attention to self-care while experiencing difficult and challenging life circumstances. Adequate sleep, healthy eating habits, and relaxation all have a direct effect on our biochemical balance and general well-being.

Yoga and meditation are exemplary tools for anyone's self-care kit. Diaphragmatic breathing and yoga postures are designed specifically to prevent life's stresses and strains from creating blockages in the body's energy systems. Yogis believe that a dedicated practice of yoga keeps the life force circulating through the body's energy centers, promoting abundant health and well-being. Simply doing things you enjoy can also directly affect the brain's chemistry. Watching a sunset, sharing a hug or a laugh with a loved one, taking in a hockey game, listening to favorite music can all improve your mood—and your health.

## Philip's Story

Philip was a busy corporate lawyer who felt consumed by his work. Phil had just made partner in a large and prestigious law firm. His habit was to work ten to twelve hours a day during the week, often without taking any time off in the day to adequately refuel his body with food. Phil's weekends were of a similar nature. Upon arising he nibbled on a muffin and ingested several cups of coffee while reading the newspaper and then was out the door to the office.

Phil said he was beginning to feel like a mole; being winter it was often already dark when Phil emerged from his office on Saturdays. Phil reported that he was plagued by headaches, a chronically sore jaw, and a mind that was constantly racing. He was having difficulty not only getting to sleep but staying asleep.

Phil said he could hardly remember how he got to this point. He had never made the conscious decision to work in a large, busy law firm. He sort of fell into it, just like he slid into the habit of working long days. Phil had been at the top of his class when he graduated from law school. He had been easily seduced by the attractive package offered him by the blue-chip law firm he had clerked for. He anticipated a life of excitement, high pay, and prestige.

Burnout and job dissatisfaction are not rare in the ranks of those who work for large organizations such as the one in which Phil worked. In our first meeting Phil provided me with an article that documented the lives of people employed in positions such as his. Alcoholism was rampant, as was divorce and family breakdown. Phil shared with me that many of his friends who had been married when they started their positions had separated from their spouses even before they had completed their third year of marriage.

Phil wanted out of the web that he had woven himself into. "I'm thirty-four years old and I want a life outside of the narrow confines of work," he declared. For him that meant the possibility of getting married, starting a family, and having leisure time to do things that gave him pleasure. Phil fairly snorted when I asked him what activities he missed taking part in. He said he really didn't have any idea anymore. "I sort of lost track of my interests in law school. But I owe myself the luxury of finding out." Phil was not certain how he would expedite the change he needed in his life, but he was certain of one thing. He was going to do it—and soon.

Phil asked that I provide him with some Yoga on the Ball stretches and tips for relaxation. Phil already owned an exercise ball. He had seen one in a store window along with a simple description of the benefits of ballwork and the notion really appealed to him. He purchased the ball that day but hadn't yet touched it—he hadn't even taken the ball out of the box and inflated it.

I started Phil with some relaxing Yoga on the Ball stretches designed to release tension and soreness from the muscles. The stretches targeted the base of the neck and moved down the body. I also gave Phil some homework that I felt would help him in his quest to unwind and have a less stressful day.

Phil was to set the mood for relaxation in his den by using the soft low lighting available there. We agreed that Phil would no longer do office work in that room. He had fallen into the habit of trying to knock off some work

while watching his favorite television programs, usually old movies. "Aahhh,"
I responded when he told me of this habit. "Here's an activity you enjoy but
don't allow yourself to fully engage in." Phil was beginning to realize that he
was doing a poor job of both relaxing *and* working when he brought work into
his den. Phil would now work at home only in the out-of-the-way room that
he had set aside as an office. In that room it was easier for Phil to remain
focused and get the work done, and thus strike that work from his to-do list
more quickly. Phil's den was to be used for recreation and relaxation only.
That way when he walked into this room his body could immediately receive
the cue that it was time to relax.

The other bit of homework that we started with was relaxation stretches.
Each night before bed Phil was to complete his repertoire of stretches. He was
to then secure his exercise ball in a corner of the den, support his feet on it,
and practice deep diaphragmatic breathing while consciously drinking in the
relaxing sensations he was experiencing. Phil got immediate satisfaction from
this nightly ritual and reported that he fell asleep much more quickly and
awakened less often during the night.

Phil began to integrate the diaphragmatic breathing into his morning
showers. He said this simple habit seemed to set his mental thermostat for the
day, helping him to remain more calm and focused. When his mind started to
race and panic began to set in Phil was to practice diaphragmatic breathing
and was to visualize himself relaxing in his den with his feet propped on the
ball. Then, before returning to the work on his desk, Phil would massage his
jaw and cheekbones as well as perform some acupressure techniques designed
specifically for stress management.

Phil describes his body's response to the techniques he was using like this.
"It takes a few minutes of concentrated attention to restore my body to 'pre-
panic mode,' but my new first-aid stress management system does work. When
I first began practicing these relaxation techniques I was employing them five
or more times a day. Now I'm down to two times a day, which seems to carry
me through the day quite well. The ball was the key to everything for me. It
started me on a different path. The unique stretching positions coupled with
the breathwork that Yoga on the Ball offered me was just what I needed. It was
comforting. It fit."

Over the course of the following weeks Phil began to talk with some of the
men and women he knew who were employed at smaller law firms. Phil soon
concluded that a smaller firm would afford him the leisure time and the
decreased stress level that he was desperately seeking. It was becoming
increasingly clear to Phil that activity was a necessity for his life. He didn't feel

that he was the type to hang out at the gym but was looking forward to working his way beyond the restorative stretches on the ball to some of the more challenging postures.

## The Costs of Stress

It is estimated that, in the United States alone, the cost to industry from stress-related illness is more than $200 billion. Stress is linked to a plethora of illnesses and conditions. Dean Ornish, M.D., is a world-renowned cardiologist credited with proving that heart disease could be reversed by eating a low-fat diet and using stress management tools such as yoga. According to Dr. Ornish more than 40 million Americans suffer from cardiovascular disease and more than 60 million have high blood pressure—and the numbers are growing. Ailments such as headaches and back pain, insomnia, asthma, allergies, diabetes, and other chronic illnesses can all be linked to stress. The breathing exercises and gentle stretches in this chapter can be quite useful in reducing the stress that leads to disease. The asanas in this chapter as well as the muscle-conditioning exercises in previous chapters are helpful for lowering cholesterol and triglycerides and will leave you less vulnerable to heart disease, diabetes, and other illnesses.

The stress reaction, once crucial to our survival, is in many cases working against us now. How often is it that we must worry about being lunch for a dinosaur? Our ancient forefathers and foremothers ran from or fought such dangers, and so their nervous systems naturally righted themselves (unless, of course, a person did become lunch!). Modern people react to modern-day stresses such as changes in job security, relationship challenges, or parenting problems with the same physiological response—the fight-or-flight reaction, which increases blood pressure, heart rate, and muscle tension and floods the body with stress-related hormones. Healing and reparation in the body are brought to a standstill.

Anything that we perceive as a stressor can bring about the body's stress response. Those who have a number of stresses and changes occurring in their lives can become stuck in this chronically elevated state of being, unable to relax or sleep well or to rid themselves of depression and agitation. People who are in this state need something to break the cycle. For Phil the breathing exercises and relaxation stretches broke the cycle of stress and panic.

The goal of restorative asanas is to bring balance and healing to the body. The stretches are designed to help squeeze toxins from the muscles, decreasing soreness and spasm. In postures where the legs are elevated heart function is enhanced as lymph, blood, and other fluids move from the lower extremities to the upper body. Spinal twists pump out tension and nourish the spinal muscles with oxygen-rich blood. The internal organs are massaged by forward bends and nourished with fresh blood by backbends. The relaxation brought about by restorative asanas and breathwork lowers heart rate and blood pressure, slows brain waves, and improves the functioning of the immune system.

## Restorative Yoga and Medical Conditions

Restorative Yoga on the Ball is appropriate for people who have fibromyalgia, arthritis, and other medical conditions that challenge one's ability to move with ease and without pain. For those with fibromyalgia many forms of exercise are too intense. Fibromyalgia sufferers spend many of their days overwhelmed with fatigue and soreness. When they have a day where they do feel as if they have some reserve energy for exercise and are not plagued by soreness it is imperative that they have a program that allows them to exercise gently and can gear their energy expenditure accordingly. Those who suffer from fibromyalgia must pace themselves—it is not reasonable to expect that a person with this condition will be able to exercise on the same day that she gets groceries or cleans the house. However, stretching can be done on a daily basis; indeed, some people with fibromyalgia find that they fare best when they stretch several times per day. The soft, cushioned surface of a partially inflated ball makes restorative stretches comfortable even for fibromyalgia sufferers, whose bodies are often sore to the touch and who consider the floor an unacceptable surface for exercise. If this is the case for you, use the ball and a thick, super-padded yoga mat for relaxing in these stretches.

Similarly, non–weight-bearing, low-impact activities are recommended for the arthritis sufferer. While other activities are too hard-driving for someone who has arthritis, the gentle restorative asanas in this chapter are often just the ticket for giving the body a chance to move without inducing lasting pain. The ball allows you to gently and slowly roll into position. If a joint's range of motion becomes too great and begins to cause pain for the exerciser, he can adjust the tension of the stretch or the positioning of his body with a simple roll of the ball.

A person who has arthritis will almost inevitably experience some degree of pain when exercising; an exercise regimen is considered to be a success if pain does not linger for two hours after exercise. Using ice or heat before and after activity can increase the comfort of the exerciser with arthritis.

People with mild multiple sclerosis can benefit from proprioception training and gentle stretches on the ball, as well, as long as they do not get too overheated. Typically a bad "spell" follows when a person with MS overexerts herself. The key here is to plan exercise so that the person with MS does not tire herself with other life activities.

Physical therapists widely use the ball with their patients. Those rehabilitating from injury and/or surgery of the lower extremities may sit on an exercise ball to limit weight bearing. In cases of injury to the upper extremities patients can perform partial weight bearing push-ups and other exercises to benefit the area by supporting the chest on the ball. In the case of a shoulder injury where the goal is to improve range of motion the ball can be rolled up and down a wall to provide muscle conditioning opportunities without overtaxing the joint. The goal in all rehabilitation is to strengthen the area of injury in a graduated and systematic fashion and to retrain proprioception. The ball is a perfect tool for meeting these goals.

## The Asanas

You do not have to be suffering from a medical condition or feel overwhelmed by stress to embrace the restoration and relaxation poses. No matter what your state, these asanas help maintain body and mind in good working order.

Move into each asana slowly and gently so that you can carefully determine what the optimal position is for your body. If you press too deeply into a stretch you will find that the muscle tightens instead of elongating. It is imperative that you pay attention to the cues that your body is giving you. Hold each posture for approximately thirty seconds. Pay attention to how a muscle feels when you are holding the stretch. You want to feel gentle tension only.

Experiment with slowly rolling and repositioning the ball with each asana so that you can target slightly different muscle fibers and stretch the muscles from various angles. The curved surface of the ball helps us to access a greater range of motion to stretch the muscles and open the joints in ways that are not possible when working on the floor.

In working with these asanas I recommend that you choose the restorative poses that feel right for your needs on any given day. Or you may wish to work with three or four restorative asanas for a week or two, then rotate to some other postures in the repertoire. (Please heed this important note: spinal twists *should not* be practiced by anyone who has undiagnosed back pain or disc injury.) Complete your relaxation with your feet resting on the ball in Shavasana and let the wavelike motion of your breath take over your body.

# Modified Fish (Matsyasana)

Fish pose stretches a number of muscle groups in the upper body and fills the lungs with oxygen; as a "body opener" it is useful in promoting relaxation. Yogic theory states that this posture stimulates the calcium-regulating parathyroid glands, situated in the neck. Adequate calcium production is essential to the health of the heart, bones, and teeth.

The traditional version of Matsyasana can place undue pressure on the cervical discs of the neck; the neck is hyperextended and the body's weight is partially supported by the head, causing damage to the spine or exacerbating pain or irritation that is already present. By executing the posture on the ball we alleviate these concerns. Range of motion with respect to the neck is naturally limited by the ball, thus the neck is not hyperextended and the ball supports the body weight so that the cervical discs are not compressed.

**Purpose** To stretch the chest and shoulders. To extend the back. To promote relaxation in the body.

**Watchpoint** • Do not overextend the neck.

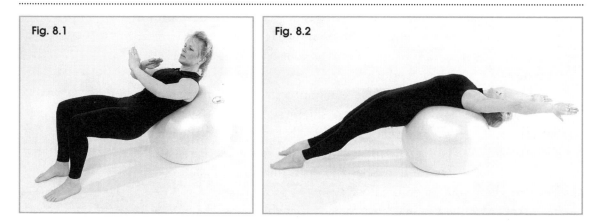

Fig. 8.1    Fig. 8.2

*starting position*

Sit in the center of your ball, feet parallel and hip-distance apart.

*movement*

**1.** Slowly walk your feet out in front of you until the upper back and shoulders are totally supported by the ball. Cross your hands at the heart (fig. 8.1). Inhale and exhale here.
**2.** Inhale as you raise your arms overhead and push into your feet to arch the body over the ball

(fig. 8.2). In this position the gentle arch in your lower back is supported by the round cushion of the ball.
**3.** Indulge in deep diaphragmatic breathing here for as long as is comfortable. Savor the release in the upper body—sometimes you can almost feel the muscles elongating fiber by fiber. Focus on sending the breath to the places in the body that require more space to decrease tightness there.
**4.** To exit the pose allow the ball to roll toward the toes as you drop your buttocks to the floor.

136

# Yoga Side Stretch

Lateral stretches can be very soothing for the spine. In yoga we often fold forward and extend backward, but we can sometimes neglect to include side stretches in our repertoire of exercises. Side stretches can help tone the oblique abdominals, muscles responsible for side bending, and maintain suppleness in the spine.

At the beginning of this stretch it is imperative to lengthen the spine first, drawing up out of the torso before moving into a side stretch. Side bends also help to move toxins out of the muscles so that prana can flow more freely up and down the spine.

**Purpose** To stretch the side of the body. To tone the oblique abdominals.

**Watchpoint** • Begin with lengthening through the spine and be sure to keep the spine lengthened through the stretch.

*starting position*

**1.** Pick up the ball and hug it to the right hip with the right hand.
**2.** Stand with the feet hip-distance apart. Find neutral spine by using the Postural Setup, paying special attention to elongating through the spine.

*movement*

**1.** Inhale.
**2.** Exhale and lift your left arm overhead as you lean to the right, stretching the left side of the body. Guide the ball down your right leg as you are leaning to the side (fig. 8.3). Hold this position for two breaths.
**3.** Straighten the spine and shift the ball so that it rests on your left hip.
**4.** Repeat on the opposite side.

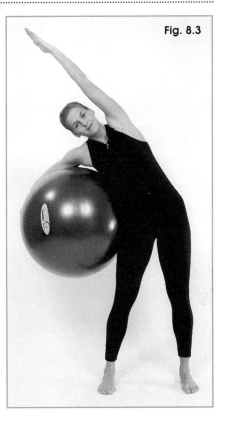

**Fig. 8.3**

137

# Standing Cat (Bidalasana)

This posture can be used to warm up the back for a gentle, stress-relieving practice. It stretches the muscles of the back and helps to create suppleness and to relieve tension.

**Purpose** To stretch the latissimus dorsi and the hamstrings. To release tension from the spine.

**Watchpoint** • Keep a slight bend in the knees throughout the asana.

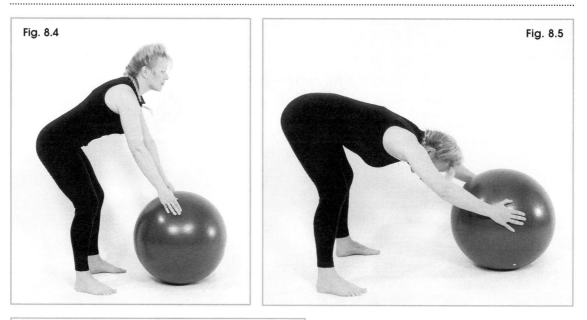

Fig. 8.4

Fig. 8.5

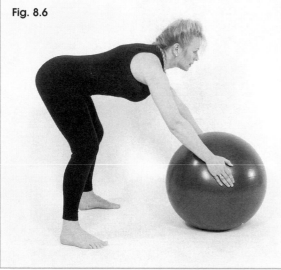

Fig. 8.6

### starting position

Stand slightly hinged at the hip joint, with the feet hip-distance apart and the ball directly in front of you, hands resting on top of the ball (fig. 8.4).

### movement

**1.** Exhale and roll the ball forward until your arms are fully outstretched. Keep the head lined up with the arms (fig. 8.5).
**2.** Inhale as you extend the spine slightly and lift the head to gently look up, keeping the hands in contact with the ball (fig. 8.6).
**3.** Repeat this movement two more times.

# Lion Pose (Simhasana)

When you practice this posture you resemble a wide-mouthed lion roaring with all its might. Lion pose is unique in that it is beneficial to areas of the body that most asanas do not address. This posture helps relieve tightness in the jaws, mouth, throat, and tongue. It is useful to those who suffer from grinding the teeth or clenching the jaw. Lion asana also stretches the tissue around the vagus nerve, the longest cranial nerve and one that works with most organs in the abdominal and thoracic cavities. The vagus nerve also connects to the pharynx, the larynx, and to glands that produce digestive juices and other secretions. It has been found that stimulation of this nerve can help to control seizures and reduce depression.

According to yogic theory the Lion asana can help to prevent or cure sore throats. It is also thought to create awareness of how prana can be directed to correct imbalances within the body. Many people suffer from tension and soreness in the jaw muscles. This is a good exercise to do several times throughout your workday to alleviate tension that can lead to stiff jaw muscles. You may find that you access the playful child within you when you practice this posture.

**Purpose** To stretch the tissues around the vagus nerve. To promote relaxation and release tension from the jaw.

**Watchpoint** • Do not open the jaw so wide that the jaw feels uncomfortable; this asana is meant to be a releasing pose.

*starting position*

Sit tall on the ball, feet parallel and shoulder-distance apart (fig. 8.7). Find neutral spine by using the Postural Setup.

*movement*

**1.** Open your jaw as wide as feels comfortable and stick your tongue out so that the tip of the tongue is pressing toward the floor (fig. 8.8).
**2.** Hold for as long as you like. Most people find that around 15 seconds is right.
**3.** Repeat one to three times.

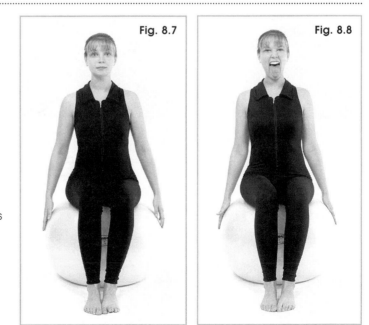

Fig. 8.7

Fig. 8.8

## Neck Stretch

Enjoy the comfort of sitting on your ball to perform this stretch but know that you can do it anywhere. This stretch provides welcome relief to sore, tired neck muscles and is useful as a preventive measure to keep muscle tension from accumulating. You may want to practice this periodically throughout your workday, as well as before bed and as part of a cooldown after a Yoga on the Ball session.

**Purpose** To rid tension from the neck by stretching the rear neck muscles.

**Watchpoints** • Do not overstretch the neck. • Do not yank on the head but rather use the hand as a gentle weight.

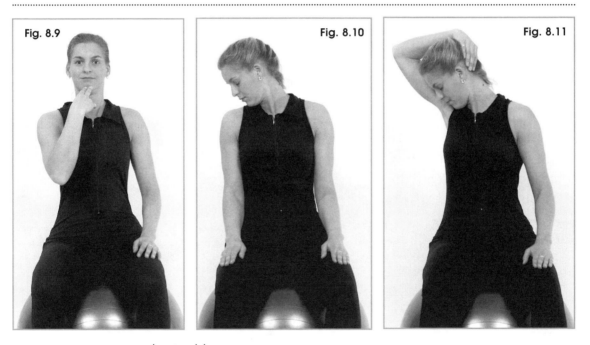

Fig. 8.9    Fig. 8.10    Fig. 8.11

### starting position

Sit tall and erect on the ball, feet parallel and shoulder-distance apart. Find neutral spine by using the Postural Setup.

### movement

**1.** Retract the chin as you do in the Postural Setup (fig. 8.9).
**2.** Turn the head gently to the right and look down at the shoulder (fig. 8.10).
**3.** Lift the right arm and cup the round part of the head at the base of the skull (fig. 8.11). Do not pull on the head. Rather, allow the hand to rest like a weight on the back of the head as you feel the muscle lengthen.
**4.** Inhale and exhale, gently adding weight through the hand to increase the stretch as you desire.
**5.** Release the arm and slowly return the head to center.
**6.** Repeat on the other side.

# Spinal Twist (Maricyasana)

This relaxing twist can be performed daily to release tension buildup in the hip and buttocks area. You will find this exercise is useful in the morning to help loosen your joints and prepare your muscles for the day ahead. It is also useful as a relaxing stretch that can be performed before bedtime to help rid your body of the tensions of the day. According to yogic teaching spinal twists help release toxins from the body so that prana can flow more freely up and down the spine.

**Purpose** To maintain unrestrained freedom of movement in the spine. To nourish the muscles and nerves along the spine.

**Watchpoints** • Be sure to keep the spine elongated throughout this asana. • Twist slowly so that you can monitor the comfort of your spine during the rotation.

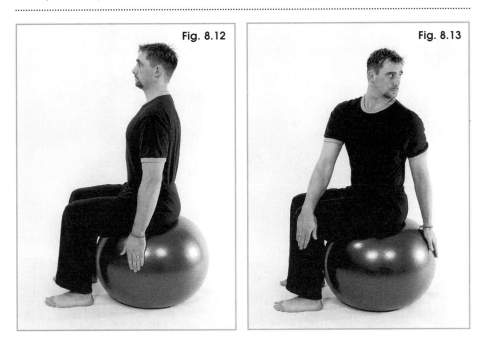

Fig. 8.12

Fig. 8.13

### starting position

Sit on the ball, feet parallel and shoulder-distance apart. Find neutral spine by using the Postural Setup (fig. 8.12).

### movement

**1.** Inhale and lengthen through the spine.
**2.** Exhale as you gently twist your spine to the left, placing your left hand behind you, palm down, and your right hand on your left leg (fig. 8.13).
**3.** Inhale and lengthen the spine.
**4.** Exhale as you gently deepen the twist, pressing the left leg to increase the rotation if you wish.
**5.** Hold the twist for three breaths.
**6.** Slowly return to the starting position.
**7.** Repeat the exercise on the opposite side.

# Kneeling Cat (Bidalasana)

This exercise is a variation of the Standing Cat pose (see page 138) and, like that version, is an effective tension-relieving warm-up for the spine. The Cat pose promotes circulation of fluid in and out of the discs between the vertebrae, helping to maintain back health. The cushioned surface of the ball makes this stretch even more enticing.

**Purpose** To release tension from the spine. To stretch the erector spinae.

**Watchpoints** • Maintain length in the spine throughout the asana. • Keep the hips aligned over the knees, as bending the knees to too great a degree can stress the knee joints.

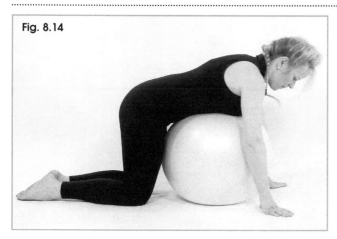

Fig. 8.14

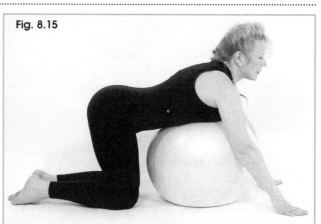

Fig. 8.15

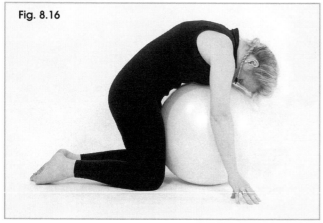

Fig. 8.16

*starting point*

Kneel on the floor over the ball, hips aligned over knees (fig. 8.14).

*movement*

**1.** Inhale as you lift the head and arch the back slightly (fig. 8.15).
**2.** Exhale as you drop the head and round the spine (fig. 8.16).
**3.** Repeat this rhythmic movement as many times as is comfortable.

## Thread the Needle

Thread the Needle is a variation of the Cat pose and usually follows Cat pose. The name of this asana comes from the threading action of the arm underneath the body. Some yoga experts believe that the phrase "thread the needle" refers to the action of filling the body with prana, or life force. This is an effective multijoint yoga stretch for relieving tension in the upper body.

**Purpose** To stretch the rear shoulders, the back, and the latissimus dorsi.

**Watchpoint** • Align the hips over the knees or just behind the knees. Bending the knees too much can stress the knee joints.

*starting position*

1. Kneel in front of your ball.
2. Place your hands on top of the ball and look down so that your head, back, and arms are aligned.
3. Press your hips back so that your hips are aligned over or slightly behind your knees (fig. 8.17).
4. Inhale and exhale here.

*movement*

1. Inhale.
2. Exhale as you take your left hand from the ball and thread it underneath your right arm (fig. 8.18).
3. Continue to actively reach across the body with your left arm, feeling the gentle release in the back of the upper body. Breathe and continue reaching in this position for as long as feels comfortable.
4. Slowly return to the starting positon, replacing the left hand on the ball.
5. Repeat on the other side.

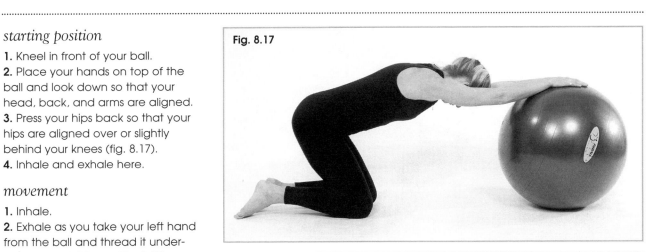

Fig. 8.17

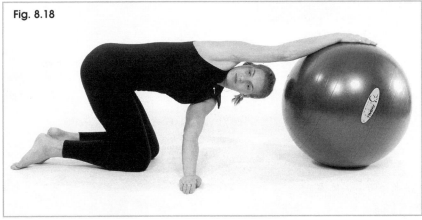

Fig. 8.18

143

# Pigeon Pose (Raja Kapotasana)

Pigeon Pose elongates the piriformis muscle. When the piriformis muscle is tight it can irritate the sciatic nerve bundle, which is situated nearby. People who drive or sit a great deal will find this stretch helpful in preventing pain and soreness.

**Purpose** To stretch the hip and release tension from the buttocks area.

**Watchpoint** • If you have any existing problem with your knees or find this that this stretch causes pain or soreness in the knees you should refrain from doing it.

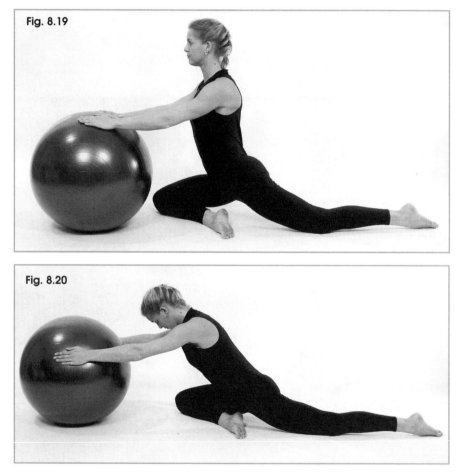

Fig. 8.19

Fig. 8.20

### starting position

**1.** Sit on the floor with the soles of the feet pointing toward one another.
**2.** Place the ball in front of you, holding it in place with your hands.

### movement—level one

**1.** Extend your left leg behind you so that the upper thigh is turned toward the floor as you simultaneously drop the right foreleg toward the floor (fig. 8.19). Position your hands on top of the ball. Feel the stretch in the buttock and hip area of the bent (right) leg.
**2.** Breathe slowly and calmly and make sure you don't hold the breath. Maintain the stretch for as long as feels comfortable.

### movement—level two

From the full extension above, roll the ball forward until the arms are fully extended in front of you (fig. 8.20). Closely monitor the stretch in the right buttock and hip. If you feel excessive discomfort in the buttocks area go back to performing the previous movement.

*movement—level three*

From the full extension above, fold forward from the hips and slowly roll the ball forward until your chest is resting on your front bent knee (fig. 8.21). Consciously monitor your comfort level and stop in the place that provides you with the amount of stretch that is comfortable for you.

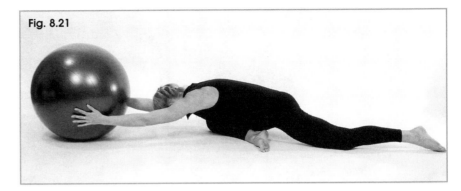

Fig. 8.21

# Reclined Hamstring Stretch (*Supta Padangusthasana*)

Tight hamstring muscles can pull the pelvis out of alignment, leading to poor posture and low-back pain. For this reason, stretching the hamstrings should be part of everyone's self-care routine. Standing hamstring stretches do not allow the muscle to completely relax, as the muscle is partially contracted in order to support the body in an upright position. Reclined Hamstring Stretch lets this important muscle group receive a full and unimpeded stretch as well as maintaining neutral spine and pelvis.

This stretch is performed with a stretch rope, a yoga belt, or a towel. It often takes at least a minute for hamstrings to relax, so be patient in this pose. Bring your attention to sending breath to the places that are tight. When my hamstring muscles are particularly tight I visualize my hamstrings as a piece of putty or chewing gum. As the muscles become warmer I imagine each fiber fluidly elongating into a full, satisfying stretch.

**Purpose** To stretch the hamstring muscles.

**Watchpoints** • Make sure that you position the rope or yoga belt so that it does not pull on the toes (which will stretch the calf muscle). You want to isolate the hamstring muscles and stretch only those muscles.

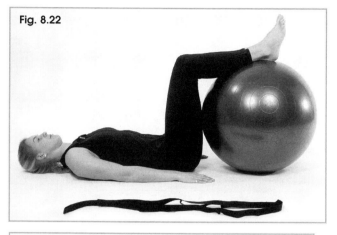

Fig. 8.22

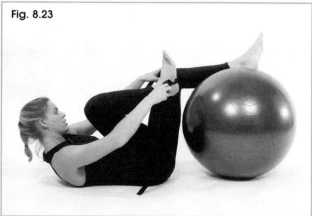

Fig. 8.23

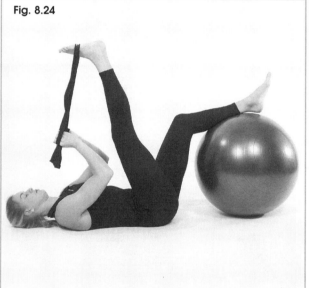

Fig. 8.24

### starting position

Lie on your back with your calves resting on the ball. Your stretch rope or towel should be accessible to you, on the floor at your side (fig. 8.22).

### movement

**1.** Sling your towel or stretch rope across the arch of the right foot (fig. 8.23).

**2.** Slowly straighten the leg, making sure the pelvis stays in contact with the floor (fig. 8.24). Be sure to keep the knee slightly bent so that you do not lock the knee joint.

**3.** Breathe deeply and rhythmically as you feel the stretch at the back of the leg. Do not allow yourself to stretch so far that you feel pulling behind the knee. Hold for as long as you are able to detect that the muscle is still stretching. Stay with it; do not release until you are certain the muscles have elongated as far as they can.

**4.** Return the leg to the ball and switch sides.

**5.** Repeat the asana once again on both sides of the body.

## Cobbler Pose (Baddha Konasana)

Cobbler pose provides an effective stretch for the muscles of the inner thigh, often a site of tight musculature, especially in men. The ball is especially useful in this pose not only because it provides support for the upper body while gravity does its work to lengthen the groin muscles but also because of its assistance in establishing the tension in the stretch. If you roll the ball toward the body and bring the heels closer to the groin you can increase your stretch. If you roll the ball away from the body you can decrease the stretch. This pose is thought to strengthen the bladder and aid in menstrual and pregnancy problems.

**Purpose** To stretch the inner thighs.

**Watchpoint** • Be careful not to force this stretch by pressing on the legs or knees; this can lead to injury. Instead, be patient in letting the muscles elongate on their own.

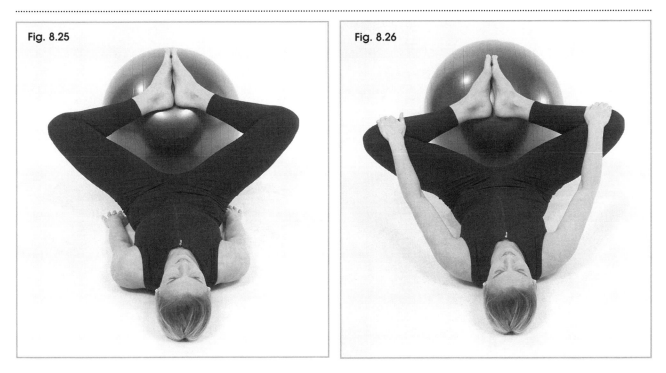

Fig. 8.25

Fig. 8.26

*starting position*

Lie on your back with the soles of the feet touching and resting on the ball. Allow the knees to gently open to the side (fig. 8.25).

*movement*

**1.** Place the hands on the knees to act as a gentle weight (fig. 8.26). Remember not to push on the knees. Rather, let gravity do its job.

**2.** Breathe in a slow, relaxed fashion.

**3.** Ease the feet toward your body as you feel the muscles relaxing into the stretch.

**4.** Release the stretch when you sense the muscles are no longer elongating.

## Reclining Spinal Twist

This exercise is useful in helping to release tension from the hip and spine area. Make sure that the hip is lined up with the shoulder at all times during this stretch. When you repeat this stretch on the opposite side of the body, reposition the hips before you drop the legs into the stretch. Yoga theory tells us that spinal twists help to free up the spine so that prana can circulate.

**Purpose** To stretch the hips and outer thigh. To release tension from the spinal muscles.

**Watchpoints** • Move slowly into this stretch. • Keep the chest oriented toward the ceiling.

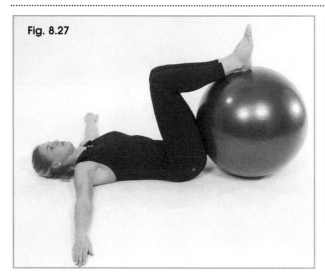

Fig. 8.27

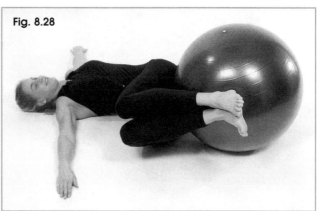

Fig. 8.28

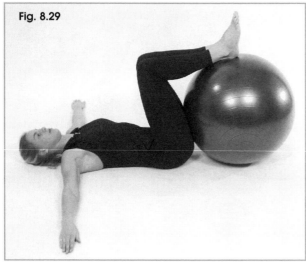

Fig. 8.29

### starting position

Lie on your back with your heels resting on the ball, knees touching and arms extending long from the shoulder joints (fig. 8.27).

### movement

**1.** Keeping the chest oriented toward the ceiling, slowly drop your knees to the right side so that they move closer to the floor (fig. 8.28).

**2.** Bring the knees back to center and repeat on the other side (fig. 8.29).

**3.** Repeat one or two more times on each side.

## Final Relaxation

Because I have practiced breathwork and meditation for many years now I am usually able to generate deep states of relaxation in a short period of time. With a regular asana practice and yogic breathing you too will learn to generate deep feelings of relaxation in your body. You may find that you become so skilled at it that you can bring about the same sorts of deep pleasure that you feel when you are appreciating a breathtaking sunset or the overwhelming beauty of the innocent look in a child's eye.

Breath is at the foundation of the movement portion of Yoga on the Ball practice. You will become increasingly aware of this as you become skilled at pairing breath with movement. The breath is also the foundation of practice in the restorative aspect of Yoga on the Ball. If you wish to meditate or commune with the Divine at the end of your practice, the next few postures will help you to prepare for that. In this segment you will want to focus closely on your breath, in this case using it as a bridge to your haven, that part deep inside you that is calm and still and as sacred as a sanctuary. The breath is the path that leads us to spirit.

When you prepare to meditate or pray you may find it helpful to focus on your breath as it moves in and out of your body, like the soothing predictability of ocean waves lapping on a beach. You may want to fix your attentions on contemplating the unity of the breath and spirit within your being. As we meditate the prefrontal lobes of the brain are charged and the limbic system, the seat of the emotions, is quieted. The pleasure centers of the brain are stimulated. Some religious and meditation experts theorize that the pleasure centers in the brain are the places where God connects with us, that in fact we are wired to be spiritual beings connected with our maker.

These next four asanas are utilized for ridding the body of tension that could preclude the practitioner from surrendering fully into a restorative state intended for mental regrouping, healing, meditation, and rejuvenation. Rocking Child Pose is an asana that may aid you in reducing muscle tightness, anxiety, or nervous energy. The rocking motion of this pose is soothing and the posture provides gentle traction and a delectable stretch for the spine. Rocking Child Pose with Massage adds the kneading of the muscles along the cervical spine to further relax the central nervous system. The Hip Lift helps reduce anxiety, as all inverted postures do; however, because this is a supported inversion there is really no work required to maintain the pose. This pose encourages blood flow to the brain, relaxing the excitable areas of the brain that need relief from swirling thought and emotion patterns. The last asana, Corpse pose, is designed to place the body in a posture known to promote deep relaxation and rest. All of these asanas, along with relaxed breathing, promote necessary balance between the sympathetic and parasympathetic components of the central nervous system.

I recommend that you choose the restorative poses that suit you on any given day. Then choose one or two postures from this final relaxation segment and finish with your feet resting on the ball. Place your hands on your belly. Focus on the breath and set sail . . . see where the breath takes you. If thoughts crowd into your awareness place them on an imaginary cloud and let them float away. Bring your awareness back to the breath. Feel deeply into the body. Let the veil between Earth and heaven slip away. Open the channels of your being to receive all that is to be received in this moment. Renew yourself by letting go.

## Rocking Child Pose

This first exercise offers the practitioner an opportunity to move in a way that inspires a sense of playfulness. Children rock naturally—from one foot to the other, back and forth on the buttocks, from heel to toe. Many times children rock when they feel anxious or upset. The ability to make this movement is a gift that we were born with and is a tool that is readily available to us; however as we mature we lose touch with many of these adaptive strategies. With this asana I invite you to surrender again into this soothing rocking motion. Remember the sense of warmth, protection, and comfort you felt when someone you loved rocked or held you as a child? As you rock on your ball call forth that comfort once again. Lose yourself in the smooth, predictable motion as you rock back and forth in this asana.

**Purpose** To release tension in the spine and the entire body.

**Watchpoint** • Keep the momentum to a magnitude that you can easily control and arrange your hands at the front of the ball so that you can stop the rocking when you wish.

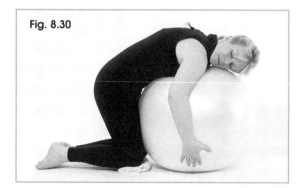

Fig. 8.30

*starting position*

Kneel on the floor and drape your body over the ball. Let your ball mould to the shape of your body (fig. 8.30). Let gravity lengthen your spine in this position. Consciously slow your breath.

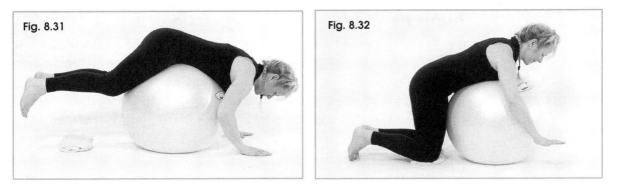

Fig. 8.31 / Fig. 8.32

*movement*

**1.** Reach your hands forward of the ball and rock onto your hands (fig. 8.31), then gently push off your hands and rock back to your feet (fig. 8.32).

**2.** Continue this rocking motion as long as you desire. Then come to rest on the ball, focusing on the lengthening of your spine and the gentle rhythm of your breath.

## Rocking Child Pose with Neck Massage

I find that it is a delicious treat to include neck massage with Rocking Child pose. I send my breath to my neck muscles as I knead the areas that still have knots.

**Purpose** To relax the muscles at the base of the skull and the neck. To maintain balance between the sympathetic and parasympathetic nervous systems.

**Watchpoints** • Be sure to place a towel under your knees if this is a tender area for you. • Do not bend your arm too much; you should feel no strain at all.

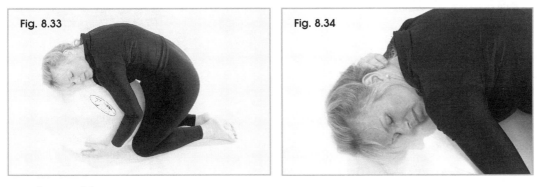

Fig. 8.33 / Fig. 8.34

*starting position*

Place the ball in front of you. You are resting on the ball with your spine curled in a C shape after having stopped the soothing motion of the Rocking Child pose (fig. 8.33).

*movement*

Lift your dominant hand and begin to massage the back of your skull and then your neck, and finish with the upper part of your back (fig. 8.34).

## Hip Lift

You may wish to use this modified inversion as a pose for meditation. Many people find that meditating in a comfortable pose is often just as beneficial, if not moreso, than having a nap. This is a rest posture that you could integrate into stressful workdays if you have a room that provides quiet. Many corporations where I have facilitated workshops have "break away" rooms that would be appropriate for this sort of rest break. Regularly practicing an asana such as Hip Lift can significantly cut your risk of stress-related diseases. Also, practicing this sort of asana as a ritual is often a good start for replacing habits that we use to help us cope with stress, such as smoking or overeating.

**Purpose** To promote relaxation and prepare for meditation.

**Watchpoints** • Move with care and control while positioning the feet on the wall. • Make sure you feel the body weight distributed between the shoulder blades, not on the neck.

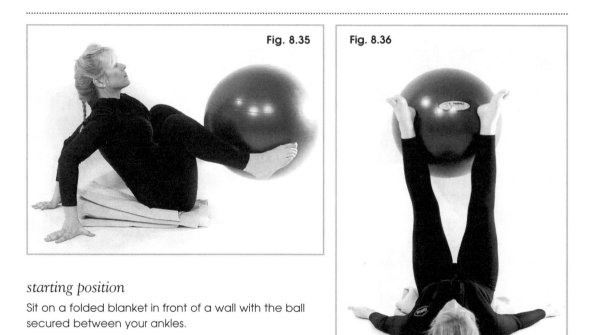

Fig. 8.35    Fig. 8.36

*starting position*

Sit on a folded blanket in front of a wall with the ball secured between your ankles.

*movement*

**1.** Rest back on your sacrum and hug the ball with your feet (fig. 8.35).
**2.** Roll the ball up the wall, coming to full extension through the legs (fig. 8.36). Scoot your hips forward toward the wall so you are in a position that gives you the desired stretch through your hamstrings. (The closer you are to the wall the greater the stretch will be.)
**3.** Rest here for as long as you want, practicing deep diaphragmatic breathing.

# Modified Corpse Pose (Shavasana)

This pose is the traditional final relaxation posture used in most classical forms of yoga. In this asana the body is to be so completely relaxed that there is complete stillness and peace and a total lack of muscle activation. Allow the muscles to release completely in this pose—after circling the feet to relieve tension allow them to splay open, toes pointing away from the body. Rest completely here for however long your schedule allows, whether five minutes or thirty. Indulge in stillness.

*movement*

**1.** Lie on the floor with your heels resting on the ball and your arms relaxed beside your body, palms down (fig. 8.37).
**2.** Make gentle circles with your heels first one way and then the opposite way before settling in and letting the feet relax.
**3.** Practice deep diaphragmatic breathing.
**4.** Rest here for as long as you like.

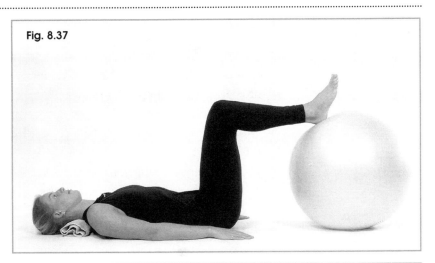

Fig. 8.37

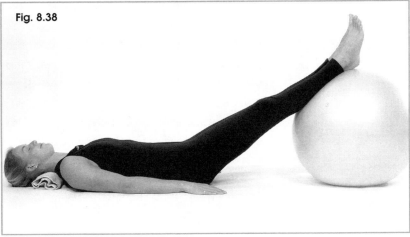

Fig. 8.38

153

## Breath and Visualization

Yoga practice begins and ends with the breath.

The following script is offered for you to use after you've practiced your final relaxation posture(s). This script can also be used as a "breather" at work or at the end of your day in preparation for a peaceful sleep. Relax deeply as you let breath move through you, knowing that the small kindnesses we gift to ourselves refuel us for carrying out the mission of our lives in grace and awareness.

1. Rest on your back, drawing your attention to the breath. Simply notice it moving in and out of your body.
2. Now observe the breath, softly and without judgment. Notice the texture of the breath: Is it short and choppy or long and calm. Are there any places in the breath exchange where the breath catches? Do you feel like you want to sigh?
3. Now focus on swelling the belly like a balloon as you inhale and flattening the belly as you exhale.
4. Focus on lengthening your respirations. Inhale and exhale to the count of ten. You may get nowhere near ten, but lengthen the respirations as fully as you can.
5. Tune in to the sensations in your mind and your body. Are your muscles relaxing? Are they feeling heavy, warm, or cool? Do you feel as if you are floating or do you have the sensation that your muscles are loose, soft, heavy, and yielding to the Mother Earth beneath you?
6. Allow your mind to become free from thought, spacious and expansive. Let your emotional being relax as you move toward tranquillity.
7. Savor any pleasant sensations you feel. Know that your bodily processes are slowing and this creates a felt sense of the body slowing down, of moving toward serenity, and creates space for healing. Know that your brain waves are slowing too, moving from beta, the attentive state in which you spend most of your waking moments, to alpha, and perhaps even to the slow delta waves in which your body can prepare for meditation.
8. Trace the path of the breath. Focus on the place where the breath enters the body. Focus on the place where it leaves the body.
9. Imagine yourself going deeper into the layers of your quiet, nourishing haven. Rest there.
10. Breathe here in this haven for five full breaths.
11. Now imagine a fresh spring breeze is entering the top of your head. Feel it brush by your cheek, blowing your hair as it enters the crown of the head.

12. Consciously slow the breath. Draw out the inhalation. Draw out the exhalation.
13. Notice the silence and stillness in the place between the breaths.
14. Know that you are creating a space for healing and wholeness in your body as you continue to enjoy long, slow, relaxed breathing. Know that you are boosting your immune system, improving the health of every cell in your body.
15. Now slowly emerge from your haven within, that quiet sanctuary.
16. Picture the number 3…
17. Picture the number 2…
18. Picture the number 1.
19. Wiggle your fingers and toes. Slowly look around.
20. Resolve to bring the experience of this tranquillity and relaxation to the regular rhythm of your life, knowing you will be healthier in mind, body, and spirit because of it. Bring the calmness of your breath into your everyday moments, knowing that life is every moment. Namaste.

# 9
# Putting It All Together

By the time you get to this chapter you have had the opportunity to practice yoga asanas appropriate for your level of conditioning and skill. Now it is important for you to link the exercises together in a way that provides you with a meaningful practice that addresses your current needs. The asana progressions outlined in this chapter will help you develop your own Yoga on the Ball practice.

In chapter 5, "Striking the Balance Between Strength and Flexibility," we discussed the importance of becoming acquainted with the idiosyncrasies of our unique and individual bodies. An important and fundamental tenet of yoga is that our earthly vehicle—the body—is to be treated like a temple. Respecting this temple means that we maintain it with proper care; to do that effectively utilizing Yoga on the Ball each person must have an understanding of her or his current fitness level. How would you characterize your current fitness status? Are you well conditioned or not at all in shape? Are you new to the practice of yoga or has yoga become a familiar friend? Are you comfortable with the level of skill you've developed with the ball or is it completely unfamiliar to you? Answering these questions will help you determine what level of practice you should begin working with.

## Your Personalized Yoga Practice

The beauty of Yoga on the Ball is that it can be tailored to fit the needs of the practitioner. Consider the introductory descriptions of each of the three levels of practice presented here and choose the one that seems right for you at this point in time. While yoga is a process, you need to find your starting point. Remember that inherent in the practice of yoga is the emphasis on present-moment experience. Please take the time to carefully consider which is the wisest starting point for you so that the practice you choose fits the level that is right for you as you are today. Embrace where you are now with no regrets about the past or compunction to jump ahead into the future. Ground yourself in the here and now and cherish what is. Whichever level you choose to begin at, the goal is to fully engage in the asanas that comprise that particular level of practice, consciously feeling each part of your body as you fully experience the asana, breathing deeply into every moment and every movement pattern.

Once you have worked your way through one level of practice presented in this chapter you will be familiar enough with that practice to further fine-tune it so that it becomes an expression of movement and presence unique to you. Pay careful attention to what you learn about your body—once you discover the muscle groups that require strengthening and rebalancing, add asanas that will support this work. Or if you find that certain of your muscle groups seem to be habitually tight, focus on carrying out the asanas that help to lengthen the muscles and free up those parts of your body. As you become proficient at the starting level of an asana introduce advanced movements to continue challenging your body and honing your present-moment mind.

Be certain to maintain that essential balance between sthira (steadiness) and sukha (comfort). I am willing to bet that there are already plenty of things in your life that you try hard to perfect. Let your Yoga on the Ball practice be a different experience. Experiment. Be playful. Approach your Yoga on the Ball practice like you are concocting a favorite tonic—choose some ingredients because they are good for you and others for the simple reason that they provide you with pleasure. After I complete a Yoga on the Ball practice I feel not only stronger and more energized but more at ease as well. I sense that I have created space in my brain as well as in the other parts of my body. I feel freer, as if the wind could blow through my body. Yogis would say that, upon completion of a vital and personalized practice, blockages in the body are cleared away and prana flows freely through each energy center, each chakra, to every part of your body.

Each Yoga on the Ball practice outlined in this chapter follows the same order: breathing and centering, postural setting, warm-up, muscle balancing asana work, balancing asanas, and relaxation/contemplation. I find it useful to begin every session with centering and breathwork in order to give me the time I need to become present in my body and create a welcome space between my last activity and the practice before me. The postural setting exercises and the warm-up prepare the body to proceed safely and less effortfully through the rest of the session. Muscle-balancing asanas strengthen and stretch the body while the balancing postures seek to improve the functioning of the core and the vestibular system. The physical balancing postures can help to balance out the emotions as well. The relaxation and restorative poses will help to further the process of balancing both the physical and emotional systems of the body.

After you choose the right starting point for your personal Yoga on the Ball practice you may wish to consider keeping notes in a journal to document your progress.

## Enhancing Your Yoga on the Ball Practice

In this section I have listed some tools that have helped me as well as my students to have an enlivened, pleasurable, and complete practice. Some of these practices may be a good fit for you too.

The first tool I want to share with you is sound, specifically incorporating music or chant into your yoga practice. Sound has the power to deeply affect our well-being. Think of the sounds that set your nerves on edge—fingernails on a chalkboard come to mind—or conversely, the sounds that relax you, like ocean waves meeting the shore. The therapeutic benefits of sound have been well documented, and research continues to be ongoing in this area. It is well accepted now that sound waves affect pulse, breathing, blood pressure, and brain waves. Therapists can manipulate sound vibrations to lower stress levels and decrease pain, and along with meditation can even bring about greater remission rates in those diagnosed with cancer. Put simply, sound can improve our mood and our health. There is even evidence to suggest that the simple act of humming or of chanting certain tones can help to improve the health of the body and the state of the mind and spirit.

Yogis have long used chant and mantra (sacred words), a practice known as naad yoga, to bring about certain desirable body and mind states. You too can enhance your state of well-being with sound. You may want to enhance your Yoga on the Ball practice by listening to instrumental selections of classical or New Age music. These types of music seem to generate the greatest healing effects. Experiment to see what musical pieces appeal to you, inviting the healing effects of sound into your practice by playing your favorite music as background. Or you may wish to incorporate other types of sound work into your practice by playing a recording of sounds such as moving water, chimes, or melodic chant. You may find that, like the yogis, you enjoy chanting or utilizing audible mantras or some other form of sound work.

The use of chant is employed by all religions and cultures, including those native to North and South America as well as Hindus, Sufis, Sikhs, Jews, Christians, and Buddists. Chanting the seed syllable "OM" is thought to bring about peace. When you chant "Hari OM" you are calling to God, the Absolute, the one who "purifies and removes all obstacles." "Hosana" is a Hebrew chant that offers up praise to God. The use of chant alters our state of consciousness to help us come into the prescence of spirit, where healing and absolute perfection abide.

The subject of sound therapy and mantra use is broad and certainly beyond the scope of this book, but if you wish to know more about the healing effects of sound you may want to consult Thomas Ashley-Farrand's book *Healing Mantras* or *The Dynamic Laws of Healing* by Catherine Ponder. Various chakra healing books discuss this topic as well.

Many yoga practitioners benefit from developing a space solely dedicated to their regular practice of yoga. Developing sacred space helps you live your life with reverence and lends depth to your practice. I like to place my exercise ball by a window so that I can look out at the trees and hear the birds singing as I practice. Reverencing nature in this way helps me to develop a state of consciousness that motivates me in my practice and keeps me anchored in present-moment awareness.

Many people do not have the luxury to devote an entire room to yoga practice space. However, designating a particular space in the room and a mat that is used only for your practice can have the same effect, helping to bring on a kind of stillness and slow, deep breathing as you settle yourself into your yoga practice space. You may find it useful to place meaningful images and other special items in this space. Some people place copies of spiritual readings in their sacred space. Prayer beads are another tool that aid the practitioner in accessing spirit. In yoga these are called mala beads; some traditions refer to them as worry beads or rosary beads. Each tradition has a slightly different way of using these beads. I find it helpful to move my fingers to a different bead each time I take a breath as I say a spiritual mantra in my head and my heart.

All of these tools can help you to prepare for your practice by inviting a positive mind state. These tools are meant to relax you and help you get in touch with your higher or spiritual self in the living space where you undertake your Yoga on the Ball practice. These tools can be useful before practicing the physical postures or even prior to relaxation or meditation.

In terms of when to practice Yoga on the Ball, there are no hard and fast rules. It is important that you pay attention to what works well for your individual needs, taking into consideration your work schedule, your energy levels, and your needs and reasons for practicing yoga. Some people find that the body accommodates best to an early morning practice; others find yoga to be a great way to settle into a good night's sleep. If your purpose for practicing Yoga on the Ball is to get into better physical shape, you may find you have more energy for that goal in the daylight hours. If you are wanting to use your practice for relaxation and rejuvenation an evening practice will be most beneficial. You may even find that you want to divide your practice into a morning and an evening session to serve both needs. This is a viable option as well.

Most important, know that less is more. Listen closely to the signs and signals your body is giving you. For instance, if your breath becomes labored slow down, or rest in Child pose. When pressing into a stretch pay close attention to the feel of the stretch to ensure that you develop gentle tension only in the targeted muscle(s) in order to get the most effective and safe results from your flexibility training. Use the sensations you are experiencing to guide you in determining how to roll the ball to intensify or to decrease the intensity of the asana or to target a slightly different muscle group. The ability to alter or change the place where you most feel the asana helps to make Yoga on the Ball a truly delicious movement practice. If you find that your form is suffering due to fatigue it is best to end your practice or to focus on the restorative aspects of practice for that day.

After you have completed the physical part of your practice you may want to enjoy a quiet meditation or prayerful communion/contemplation. A regular meditation practice helps us to develop equanimity, an inner spaciousness that allows us to be at peace in all circumstances. A state of equanimity is easier than being witness to the transient and sometimes chaotic emotions that pull us into the vortex of difficult responses to the challenges of our lives. When we have equanimity we can choose a calm response to the situation at hand.

Meditation, prayer, and quiet reflection have significant positive effects on health. In his best-selling book *Prayer Is Good Medicine* Larry Dossey, M.D., scientifically documents the miraculous medicinal effects that prayer can have on us as well as on the people and circumstances around us. Yogis have known for thousands of years that communion with the Divine brings wholeness, enlightened perspective, and meaning to existence as well as healing and a sense of connection to the self and loved ones.

The final and summary note in all these suggestions is to allow your Yoga on the Ball practice to meet you where you are. You are who you are because of where you have been, and your life experiences thus far have sown the seeds necessary to provide you with the lessons that were meant to shape the unique life force housed within your body. So wherever you are in your life is exactly where you need to be at this moment. The noncompetitive and functional practice of Yoga on the Ball is one of the tools that can help you to make manifest your unique life's potential in terms of your physical wellness, your mental clarity, and perhaps even your spiritual openness. Yogis originally used their practice to help them prepare the mind and body to commune with the Divine.

There are many who feel that cultivating a spiritual life and being in touch with a higher intelligence is the most effective way to glean information about one's true purpose in life. When we have an understanding of our true purpose we are on the way to manifesting our potential and our ultimate destiny. When we align ourselves with a higher intelligence or our highest self we make better decisions and impact on the world in a more powerful and positive way.

There are many paths leading to the sacred, and it matters not whether you are Muslim, Buddhist, Hindu, or Christian—when Spirit is housed in the temple of your being your whole life can be lived like a prayer. When we learn to live the true essence of yoga we can fortify our ties to ourselves, our neighbors, and as Swami Vivekananda did back at the turn of the twentieth century, between entire nations. We can learn to transcend our differences and embrace our commonalities. Yoga helps us to transform ourselves, starting with the inner parts of our being and working toward the outer parts. Cultivate an understanding that the real essence of yoga doesn't come through while you are on the ball or the yoga mat. Rather, the spiritual power of your yoga practice shows itself in your relationships with family and friends and in your ability to honor self and others. The physical and mental power of yoga is demonstrated in improved comfort and function in activities of everyday living relevant to your own lifestyle.

Allow your Yoga on the Ball program to develop into what you need it to be, whether that be improved physical or mental adaptation or increased spiritual sensibility. Martha Graham, a pioneering modern dancer, often told her students that every person's job in life is to do everything possible to nurture the life force within so that their unique potential can fully actualize. I couldn't agree more. Allow your Yoga on the Ball practice to help you do just that—let it take the shape it needs to maintain the temple of your body and develop the unique life energy that is you.

161

The three practices that follow have been delineated by level. Page numbers allow you to cross-reference back to full instructions in the text; the photographs provide a quick visual reference.

## Level I Practice

This first-level practice is intended to give a gentle entry into Yoga on the Ball to people who have been injured and have been through active rehabilitation with a physical therapist or other physio specialist. Check with your health care provider to make sure that he or she thinks you are "exercise ready" before you begin this practice, and take great care to perform all movements slowly and with control, being certain to work with good posture and neutral alignment in every joint.

The first-level practice is also appropriate for managing stress. If you're in need of this kind of practice, choose a movement pace that fits well for your mood and encourages you to deeply immerse yourself in your sensations. Concentrate on working with the breath, breathing as deeply and slowly as you can while you mindfully making your way through the postures. Finish your practice with the visualization on page 154.

Modify any of the poses as needed to address your particular situation. This is a practice you can undertake daily.

*Breath Check*
*(p. 24)*

**1. breath check**

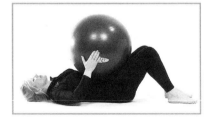

*Diaphragmatic Breathing*
*(p. 25)*

**2. diaphragmatic breathing**

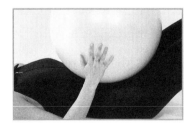

*Postural Setup: Ideal*
*Alignment (p. 38)*

**3. finding ideal alignment**

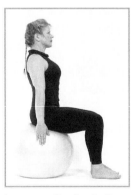

(move methodically through the steps of this postural exploration to come into neutral spine)

## *Prayer Breath (p. 28)*
**4. prayer breath**

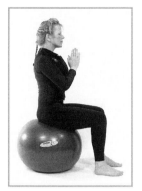

## *Prana Power (p. 27)*
**5. prana power**

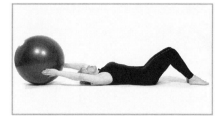

(use Prayer Breath and Prana Power as your warm-up for Level I practice)

## *Modified Fish (p. 136)*
**6. modified fish**

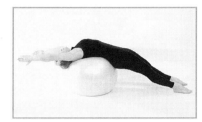

## *Lion Pose (p. 139)*
**7. lion**

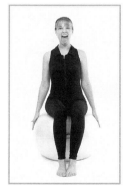

## *Neck Stretch (p. 140)*
**8. neck stretch**

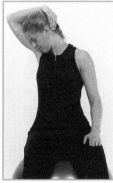

## *Spinal Twist (p. 141)*
**9. spinal twist**

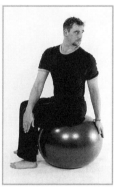

(don't include this asana in your practice if you are recovering from a spinal or disc injury)

## *Knee Lift (p. 95)*
**10. knee lift**

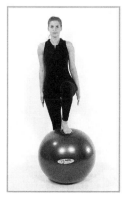

## *Tree Pose (p. 97)*
**11. tree—level one**

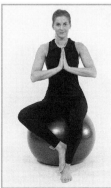

## *Thread the Needle (p. 143)*
**12. thread the needle**

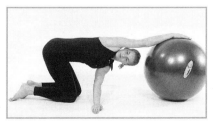

*Pigeon Pose*
*(p. 144)*

**13. pigeon pose—level two**

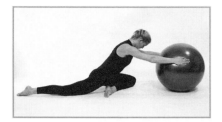

*Reclined Hamstring Stretch*
*(p. 145)*

**14. hamstring stretch**

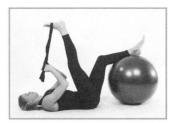

*Cobbler Pose*
*(p. 146)*

**15. cobbler pose**

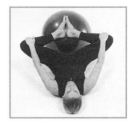

*Hip Lift*
*(p. 152)*

**16. hip lift**

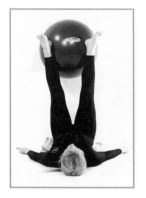

*Rocking Child Pose with*
*Neck Massage (p. 151)*

**17. child pose with massage**

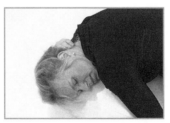

*Modified Corpse Pose*
*(p. 153)*

**18. corpse pose (fig 8.38)**

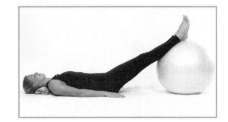

## Level II Practice

The second-level Yoga on the Ball practice is designed to fit the person who has no injuries or special medical conditions that require treatment or that could be made worse from exercise. In this basic routine concentrate on completing the movement patterns with precision and control until you can manage the posture with ease. Practice each asana slowly and carefully until you understand each step. Attempt to breathe deeply and slowly, using the breath pattern described in the directions for each asana.

This complete repertoire of exercises will address every area of the body. Practice three to five times a week to build strong, lean muscles and endurance.

*Breath Check*
*(p. 24)*

**1. breath check**

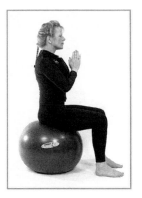

*Diaphragmatic Breathing*
*(p. 25)*

**2. diaphragmatic breathing**

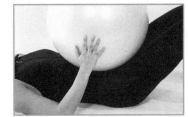

*Postural Setup: Ideal*
*Alignment (p. 38)*

**3. finding ideal alignment**

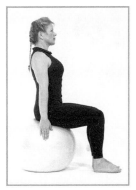

(move methodically through the steps of this postural exploration to come into neutral spine)

*Prayer Breath (p. 28)*

**4. prayer breath**

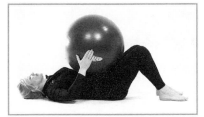

*Prana Power (p. 27)*

**5. prana power**

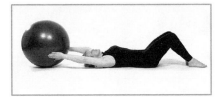

## *Sun Salutation (p. 48)*

### 6. sun salutation basic movements

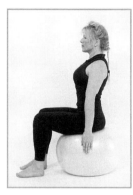
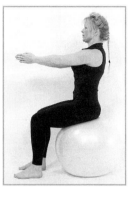
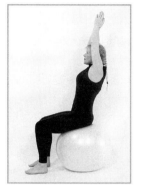
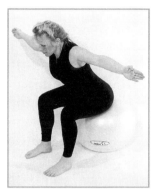

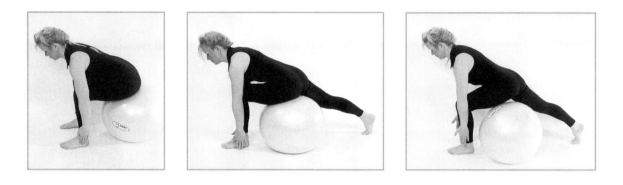

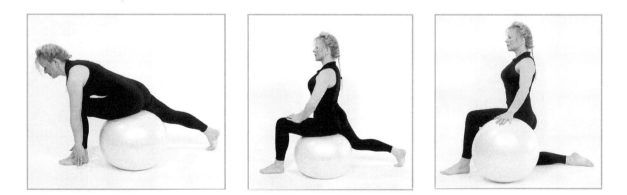

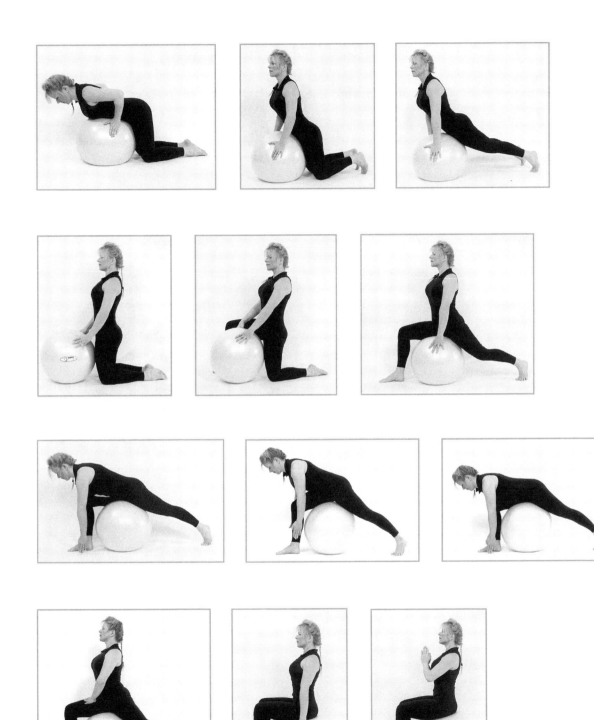

## Standing Forward Fold (p. 59)

**7. standing forward fold**

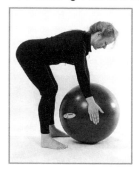

## Seated Forward Fold (p. 61)

**8. seated forward fold**

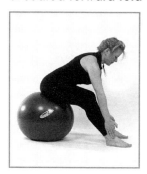

## Cobra (p. 62)

**9. cobra—level one**

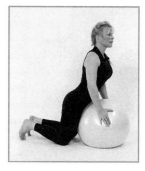

## Down Dog (p. 64)

**10. down dog**

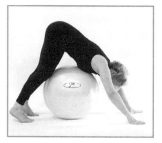

## Camel (p. 68)

**11. camel**

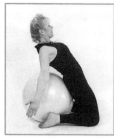

## Boat Pose (p. 80)

**12. boat—level one**

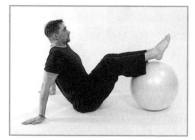

(if you can manage not to overarch the back, go to level two)

## Reverse Plank (p. 66)

**13. reverse plank—level one**

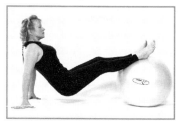

## Warrior 1 (p. 84)

**14. warrior 1—level one**

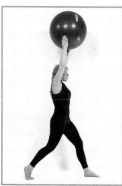

(you can substitute Chair pose (p. 71) at this point as both work the quadriceps)

## Side Plank (p. 100)

**15. side plank**

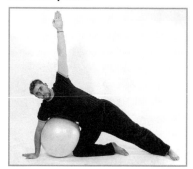

*Tree Pose*
*(p. 97)*

**16. tree—level two**

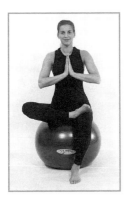

*Warrior 1 with Prayer*
*Twist (p. 89)*

**17. warrior 1 with prayer twist**

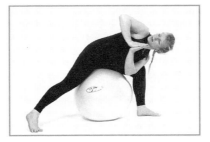

*Rocking Child Pose*
*(p. 150)*

**18. rocking child pose**

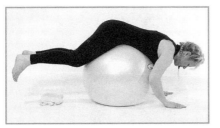

*Rocking Child Pose with*
*Neck Massage (p. 151)*

**19. child pose with massage**

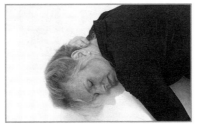

*Modified Corpse Pose (p. 153)*

**20. corpse pose**

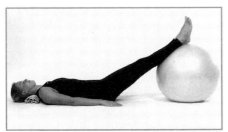

## Level III Practice

This practice is for those who have a good understanding of yoga asanas and feel confident in their skills working with an exercise ball. Athletes, yoga practitioners, and advanced exercisers who have mastered the second-level practice can move on to this sequence for a further challenge.

Working with precision and control is of utmost importance. You can "load in" versions of various postures from the Advanced Postures chapter when you're ready. Let me reiterate that it is important to first understand the mechanics of each posture before adding add the breath rhythms outlined in the instructions for each asana. This sequence can be performed three to five times per week.

*Breath Check (p. 24)*

**1. breath check**

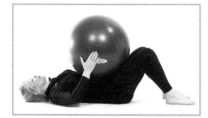

*Diaphragmatic Breathing (p. 25)*

**2. diaphragmatic breathing**

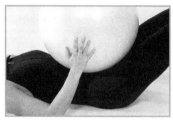

*Postural Setup: Ideal Alignment (p. 38)*

**3. finding ideal alignment**

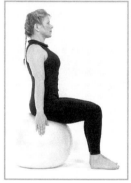

(move methodically through the steps of this postural exploration to come into neutral spine)

*Prayer Breath (p. 28)*

**4. prayer breath**

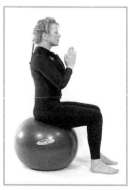

*Prana Power (p. 27)*

**5. prana power**

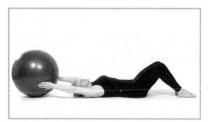

## *Sun Salutation (p. 48)*

**6. sun salutation—all movements**

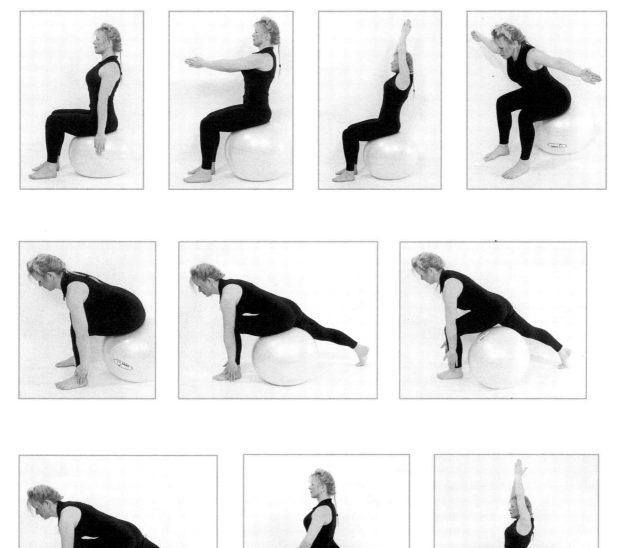

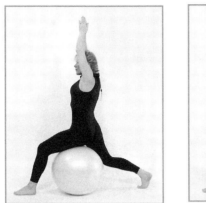 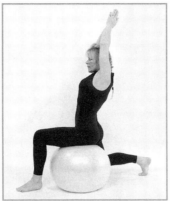 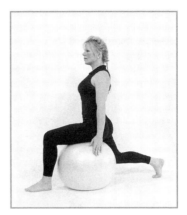

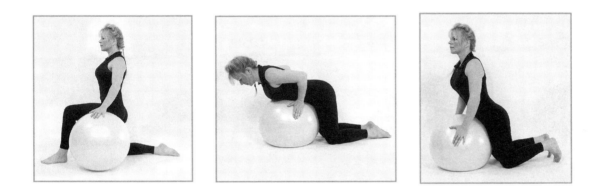

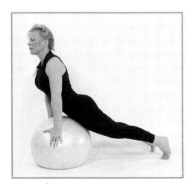 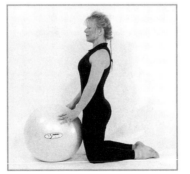 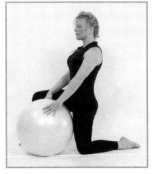

Extendsion

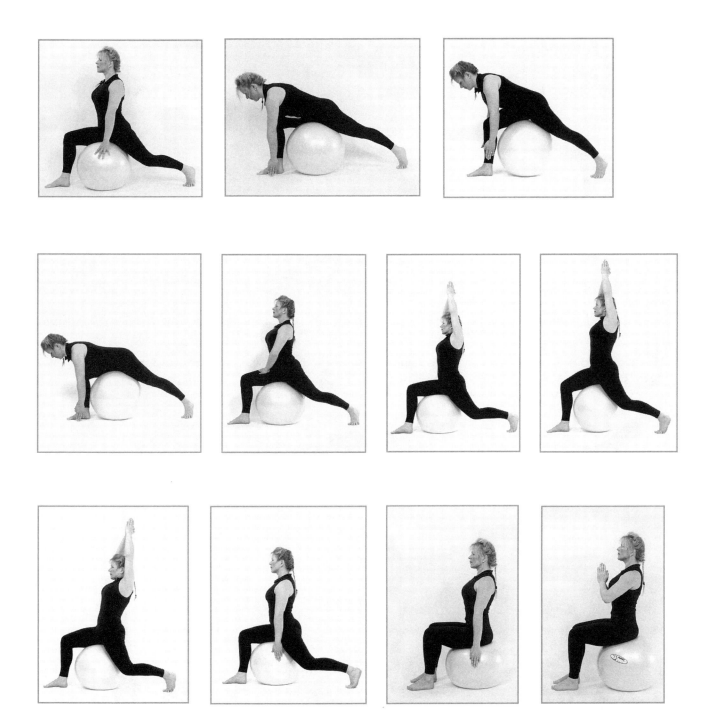

*Standing Forward Fold*
*(p. 59)*

**7. standing forward fold**

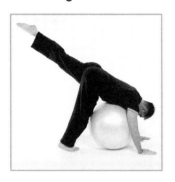

*Standing Cat*
*(p. 138)*

**8. standing cat**

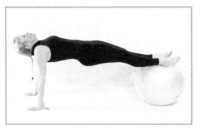

*Cobra*
*(p. 64)*

**9. cobra—level two**

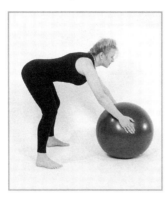

*Advanced Down Dog*
*(p. 125)*

**10. advanced
down dog**

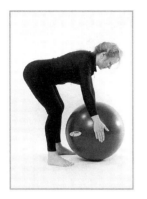

*Reverse Plank*
*(p. 66)*

**11. reverse plank—
level two**

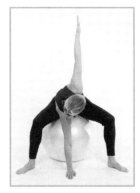

*Forward Fold with Spinal
Twist (p. 69)*

**12. forward fold with
spinal twist**

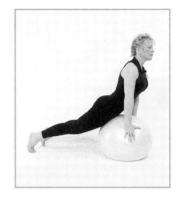

*Crow Pose (p. 75)*

**13. crow pose—level two**

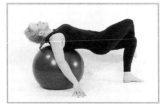

*Bow Pose (p. 73)*

**14. bow**

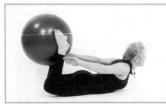

*Warrior 2 (p. 86)*

**15. warrior 2**

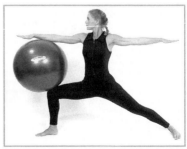

### Side-Lying Plank (p. 121)

**16. side-lying plank—level two**

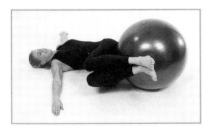

### Bridge Pose (p. 82)

**17. bridge—level two**

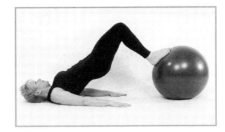

### Tree Pose (p. 97)

**18. tree—level three**

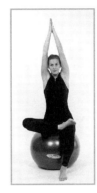

### Half Moon (p. 101)

**19. half moon—level two**

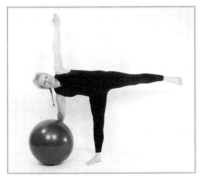

### King Dancer (p. 104)

**20. king dancer—level two**

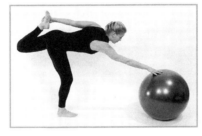

### Modified Fish (p. 136)

**21. modified fish**

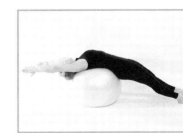

### Reclining Spinal Twist (p. 148)

**22. reclining spinal twist**

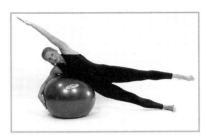

### Rocking Child Pose (p. 150)

**23. rocking child pose**

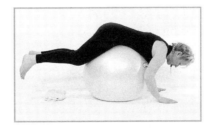

### Modified Corpse Pose (p. 153)

**24. corpse pose**

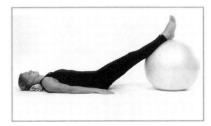

# Appendix

*Major Muscles and Their Functions*

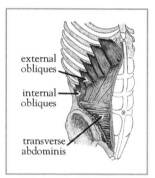

external obliques

internal obliques

transverse abdominis

## Abdominals (transverse abdominis, internal obliques, external obliques)

The transverse abdominis muscle is the deepest of the abdominal muscles. It cinches the waist and thus forms a natural corset that protects the spine; this stabilizes the columnar shape of the spine. The bracing action of the transverse abdominis helps to hold the discs in optimal alignment so that pressure is equalized throughout the spine when you bear weight. The obliques run diagonally down the sides of the waist and are responsible for the rotating and sidebending motions of the spine.

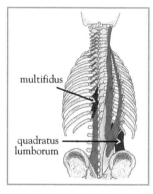

multifidus

quadratus lumborum

## Core-stabilizing triad (transverse abdominis, multifidi, quadratus lumborum)

The transverse abdominis muscle, the deepest of the abdominal muscles, forms a natural corset that protects the spine (see above). The multifidi and quadratus lumborum are the innermost muscles of the back, closest to the spine. Deep and tight up against all of the vertebrae we find the multifidi running the entire length of the spine, while the quadratus lumborum runs from the iliac crest (the top of the pelvis) to the twelfth rib. These three muscles work together to stabilize the spinal structure and protect the spine from injury during movement.

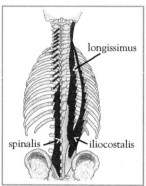

longissimus

spinalis

iliocostalis

## Erector spinae (longissimus, spinalis, iliocostalis)

The erector spinae muscles run the entire length of the spine along the vertebral column. This large mass of muscle divides and attaches in an overlapping fashion throughout the length of the spine. These muscles are responsible for pulling you back up to a standing position after you bend over to tie your shoe. The erector spinae are strengthened in Yoga on the Ball asanas when you return to an upright position following a forward bend.

### Rhomboids (rhomboid major and rhomboid minor)

These small retangular-shaped muscles extend from the spine to the scapula, attaching to the back of the shoulder blade. Their job is to draw the shoulder blades toward the spine; these muscles are important for maintaining good posture. The rhomboids are weak and overstretched in many people. You can help to keep the rhomboid muscles toned by engaging them to maintain scapular stabilization, as required in Yoga on the Ball practice.

### Latissimus dorsi

The latissimus dorsi, the largest muscle of the back, extends from the back of the pelvis to the bottom of the shoulder blades, wrapping around the ribs and attaching to the medial side of the humerus. The lattisimus lowers the arm from the front or side of the body back to the trunk and rotates the arm and shoulder inward and downward. The "lats" need to be strong in individuals who enjoy sports like canoeing or rowing, due to the repetitive motion of pulling down and back.

### Trapezius

The trapezius muscle is a large kite-shaped muscle that attaches at the vertebrae from the base of the skull and runs approximately two-thirds of the way down the back. This muscle is divided into three parts and is responsible for lifting and lowering the scapulae and drawing the scapulae closer to the spine. The trapezius can also draw the head back and sidebend or rotate the head. We require good tone in this muscle to be able to stabilize the head and scapulae in a neutral position during Yoga on the Ball practice.

### Pectorals (pectoralis major and minor)

The pectoral muscles are located in the front of the chest and under the breasts. They originate on the clavicle (collarbone), sternum, and ribs and insert on the upper part of the humerus. These muscles draw the arms across the chest, inwardly rotate the arms, and flex and extend the shoulders. It is important to stretch these muscles frequently as they become shortened in people who spend a lot of time hunched over a desk or a steering wheel.

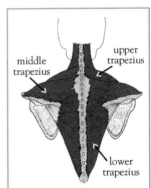

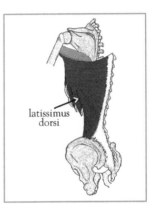

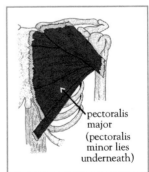

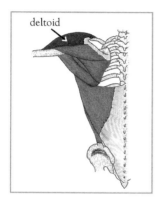

## Deltoids

The shoulder muscles consisting of the anterior, medial, and posterior deltoid wrap completely around the top of the arm. The deltoids helps to rotate the arm inward and outward and raise the arm in front, behind, and to the sides of the body. The deltoids also assist in rotating the arm inward and away from the body. The deltoids are strengthened when they assist with Yoga on the Ball movements such as raising the arms overhead in Tree pose or Chair posture.

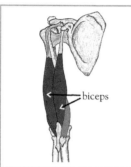

## Biceps

The bicep muscles originate at the top of the shoulder joint and attach into the forearm. Their job is to bend the arm. You use these muscles when you draw the arms into prayer position or when you bend the arms to pull the ball closer to the body when altering intensity or entering or exiting a pose. Strong biceps ease the work of lifting loads such as groceries or books, or picking up a baby.

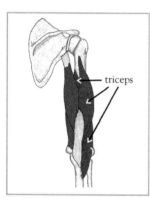

## Triceps

The tricep muscle has three distinct segments, the longest of which attaches to the scapula; the other two segments attach to the back of the humerus and run down the back of the lower arm. The triceps straighten the elbow. You strengthen these muscles in Yoga on the Ball practice when you press up into Cobra pose, a back extension, or a plank position. Toned triceps give the back of the arm a sculpted look.

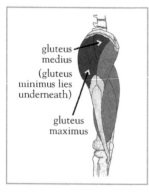

## Gluteals (gluteus maximus, gluteus minimus, gluteus medias)

The gluteal muscles are powerful movers of the hip; together the three gluteals give shape to the buttocks. The gluteus maximus, the largest muscle in the body, extends and externally rotates the thigh. The underlying gluteal medius and minimus work together to abduct and internally rotate the femur (the thighbone). We rely on our "glutes" to help us stand up, climb stairs, and jump. Hockey players rely on this "push-off" musculature, which is responsible for powerful and rapid forward skating strokes. Locust pose strengthens the gluteals.

## Hip flexors (psoas major, psoas minor, iliacus, rectus femoris)

The psoas muscles and the iliacus originate from the five lumbar vertebrae and attach on the femur. The rectus femoris, one of four muscles comprising the quadriceps group, originates on the front part of the lower pelvis and attaches onto the front of the thigh by way of the quadriceps tendon. These muscles act together to lift the leg in front of the body. These typically strong muscles become tight from frequent sitting and thus require regular stretching.

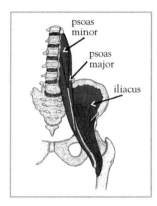

## Quadriceps (vastus lateralis, vastus intermedius, vastus medialis, rectus femoris)

For most people the quadriceps are the strongest muscles in the body. This musculature, situated at the front of the thigh, straightens the leg at the knee joint and bends the thigh at the hip. The quadricep group is strengthened in lunge positions, such as in Warrior 1. Strong quadricep muscles help to prevent knee problems and are required for activities such as walking, running, climbing, skiing, and cycling.

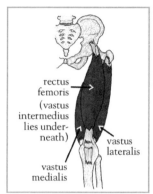

## Adductors (adductor longus, adductor magnus, adductor brevis, pectineus, gracilis)

The inner thigh muscles stretch from the pubic bone to the femur. The job of the adductors is to draw the legs in closer to the midline of the body, as when kicking a soccer ball. If these muscles become shortened due to frequent use, knee and back problems can result from the adductors pulling the femur in and the pelvis down when the body is in motion. Keep these muscles well stretched.

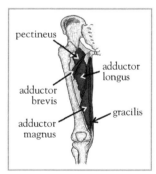

## Hamstrings (biceps femoris, semitendinosus, semimembranosus)

The hamstring group comprises the majority of muscle mass at the back of the thigh. This muscle group acts to extend the hip joint and flex the knee. The Warrior 1 lunge as well as the Bow and Locust poses strengthen the hamstrings. Since this muscle group is prone to injury through "hamstring pulls" it is wise to warm them well prior to activity and to maintain their flexibility.

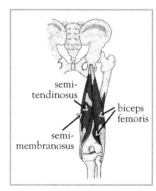

179

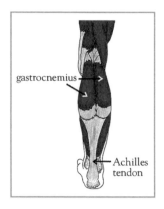

### Gastrocnemius, Achilles tendon

The gastrocnemius is the muscle that gives shape to the calves. The Achilles tendon joins the gastrocnemius (and the soleus, which lies underneath the gastrocnemius) to the heel bone. Typically the "gastrocs" are strong because they are used in walking and standing; this muscle is usually tight in women who wear high heels. The gastrocnemius muscle benefits from regular flexibility training. The Down Dog posture stretches the gastrocnemius.

# Resources

## Books

Carrière, Beate. *The Swiss Ball: Theory, Basic Exercises, and Clinical Application*. Germany: Springer-Verlag, 1998.

Coulter, H. David. *Anatomy of Hatha Yoga*. Honesdale, Pa.: Body and Breath Inc., 2001.

Craig, Colleen. *Pilates on the Ball*. Rochester, Vt.: Healing Arts Press, 2001.

Jemmett, Rick. *Spinal Stabilization: The New Science of Back Pain*. Halifax: RMJ Fitness and Rehabilitation Consultants, 2002.

Kendall, Florence, and Elizabeth McCreary. *Muscles—Testing and Function*. Baltimore, Md.: Williams and Wilkins, 1983.

Khalsa, Dharma Singh, M.D. *Meditation As Medicine: Activate the Power of Your Healing Source*. New York: Pocketbooks, 2001.

Lasater, Judith. *Relax and Renew*. Berkeley: Rodmell Press, 1995.

Cotton, Richard, ed. *Personal Trainer Manual*. (2nd ed.). San Diego: American Council on Exercise, 1996.

Posner-Mayer, Joanne. *Swiss Ball Applications for Orthopedic and Sports Medicine*. Longmont, Colo.: Ball Dynamics Inernational, 1995.

Richardson, Carolyn, Gwendolen Jull, Julie Hides, and Paul Hodges. *Therapeutic Exercise for Spinal Segmental Stabilization in Low Back Pain*. London: Churchill Livingstone, 1999.

Stark, Steven D. *The Stark Reality of Stretching*. Richmond, B.C.: The Stark Reality Corp., 1997.

Usatine, Richard, M.D., and Payne, Larry, Ph.D. *Yoga Rx*. New York: Broadway Books, 2002.

## Videos

*Colleen Craig's On the Ball: An Innovative Ball Video Based on the Work of Joseph Pilates*, VHS/color/45 mins.

*Fitball Yoga* by Carol Mitchell, VHS/color/46 mins.

*Fitball—Back to Functional Movement* by Trish Scott, VHS/color/30 mins.

*Fitball—Upper Body Challenge; Fitball—Lower Body Challenge* by Cheryl Soleway, VHS/color/45 mins. each.

*Swiss Ball Applications for Orthopedic and Sports Medicine* by Joanne Posner-Mayer, VHS/color/90 mins.

# Ball and Video Ordering Information

**Ball Dynamics International, Inc.**
Makers of Fitball®.
Catalog of exercise balls,
videotapes, and accessories.
800-752-2255.
www.fitball.com

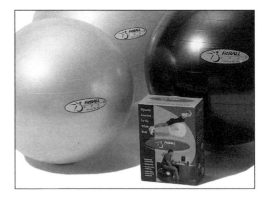

**Know Your Body Best**
Canadian distributor of
exercise balls, *Colleen Craig's
On the Ball* videotape,
therapeutic massage
equipment and supplies.
800-881-1681 (in Canada).
www.knowyourbodybest.com

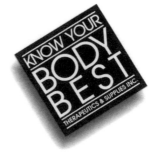

**The International Society of Yoga Education** offers yoga certification, Yoga on the Ball workshops and instructor training, and educational yoga videos and manuals. 1-877-407-YOGA (9642). www.internationalyogasociety.com

# Acknowledgments

I would like to thank my parents, Jean and Glen Gilbert, for teaching by example. As a child I learned so much about the great value and honor in hard work and simplicity in life. I cannot help but think of the Zen proverb "before enlightenment, chop wood, carry water . . . after enlightenment, chop wood, carry water." This proverb reflects the wisdom my parents imparted by example. I learned as a young child that some of the greatest lessons relevant to one's spiritual path can be found in everyday life. I still have very clear images of my father in my mind's eye—the quiet contentment in his face as he raked the yard or watched a handful of soil slowly sift through his fingers to return to the earth. My parents didn't talk much about values, they just quietly lived them, day after day.

Thank you to my mother-in-law, Gertrude Mitchell, for being an enthusiastic cheerleader in my corner at all times, and for providing practical support of babysitting and running errands for our young family during the writing of this book.

A salute to my husband, Bruce Mitchell. You are so solid. I thank you for your steadfastness, sense of humor, and practical suggestions not only during the writing of this manuscript but in the daily adventure of our lives together.

Heartfelt thank-yous to three of the great blessings in my life: my son, Dylan, and my two daughters, Savannah and Abilene. I so appreciated your selflessness and maturity in letting me have my quiet time to write. Thanks also for expressing your sincere sentimentalities on a regular basis. I learn so much from you about living yoga every day of our lives together.

Thank you to my maternal grandmother, Ethel Wittick Bonnett, who taught me as a child to count my blessings daily as we breathed calmly into the morning, kneading the bread we would bake for the evening's supper.

I was blessed to have had the expertise of my esteemed editor, Susan

Davidson. I can only believe that it was the exquisite work of the Divine that paired our energies. Her extensive knowledge of this field, her conscientiousness, and her commitment to excellence were a tremendous blessing to me. Her ability to hold the big picture together while attending to the many and varied fine details of a project of this magnitude is to be truly applauded. I will be forever grateful for her sincere and heartfelt desire to gain a thorough understanding of the vision I had for this book and for the support, sensitivity, and dedication she gave that enabled me to manifest that vision. I felt at times as if she was not only guiding my hand but holding it too, as she pointed the way to the finish line. I have great respect for Susan's outstanding skill, knowledge, and experience, and for who she is as a person as well. She truly inspired my work. With my hand on my heart, I bow to you. Namaste Susan.

I tip my hat to publisher Ehud Sperling. I am grateful for your faith in this project and for the excellence demonstrated by the entire team of players at Healing Arts Press that helped to bring this book into being. I thank Peri Champine, art director at Healing Arts Press, for creating the exquisite cover, and Jeanie Levitan, managing editor, for her warm, nurturing spirit. Thank you to Sandy Brown and Burma Cassidy for the nourishing meals and conversation shared during my stay in Vermont. I extend my appreciation to all in the friendly town of Rochester who made me feel so welcome while I was working with my editor in Vermont.

I am so very grateful to sponsor Dayna Gutru at Ball Dynamics, USA, for her gracious emotional and financial support of my work. Thank you to Joan Cofell and her son, Dana, for the tender loving care and conscientiousness in the handling of the immense photographic work involved in this project. Many thanks to Monique Haan, Todd Wood, and Sarah Hall for allowing me to use the exquisite photos of you in this book. Thanks also to Jill Ellis for the skill and effort put into developing the diagrams in the book. Thank you to Judy Watson for her many episodes of working into the wee hours of the night to place the symbols and codes in the manuscript. Thank you to Sandra Rader for the early morning hair appointments and warm words of encouragement prior to the photo shoots.

Thank you, Marion McHugh, for encouraging me to take on this project and for the warm inspirational messages that found their way from your heart to my heart during the entire writing of this manuscript. I would like to thank Sarah Hall, my assistant, for her professionalism and enthusiasm and her ability to keep things running smoothly in my office when I was knee-deep in writing. Thank you to Trish Scott for her professional opinions and uplifting humor, ever present even in the heaviest of work demands and schedules. I am grateful to Colleen Craig for leading the way with her superb work in *Pilates on the Ball*.

Thank you to Sister Dominica for encouraging me to find my own spiritual path. Thank you to Sister Sheila and various members of the Islam, Sufi, Bhuddist, Muslim, and other faiths who have shared their visions with me to encourage me to find and celebrate the oneness of all faiths committed to honoring the Divine.

Charlene Bedford, thank you for being an example of excellence and for overseeing every detail, great and small, in our office, and for your heartfelt enthusiasm and support during the writing of *Yoga on the Ball*. Thank you also to Tamar Malic for sharing your passionate, loving, and energetic spirit with our children during the busy moments of my life.

I am grateful for those who have inspired me with their commitment to excellence in their work: Mary Sanders, for her research in the area of exercise science; Donna Farhi, Judith Lasater, Dr. Richard Usatine, David Coulter, Dr. Dharma Singh Khalsa, Rachel Schaeffer, Silva Mira, and Shyam Mehta for their outstanding contributions toward making the gift of yoga accessible to all populations; and Tom Pervis, Joanne Posner-Mayer, Florence Kendall, and Dr. Steven Stark in the areas of sports medicine. Thank you to Nancy Adams, physiotherapist at the Fowler Kennedy Sports Clinic, and to Dr. Rhan Bohunicky for so kindly making yourselves available to me to answer my many and varied questions. I would like to express my sincere appreciation to the physiotherapists, sports medicine physicians, and fellow yoga instructors who have shared their expertise with me over the years and are too modest to be cited here.

Thank you to the students and instructors I train from whom I learn so much. To those of you who have let me tell your stories in this book, heartfelt thanks for sharing yourself this way. Thank you to the organizations, wellness centers, and yoga and health studios around the world who sponsor my workshops and instructor trainings. Finally, thank you to the board and faculty members of the International Society of Yoga Education for your support, encouragement, and sanctioning of my work.

# Books of Related Interest

**Pilates on the Ball**
The World's Most Popular Workout Using the Exercise Ball
*by Colleen Craig*

**Pilates on the Ball**
A Comprehensive Book and DVD Workout
*by Colleen Craig*

**Abs on the Ball**
A Pilates Approach to Building Superb Abdominals
*by Colleen Craig*

**Body Rolling**
An Experiential Approach to Complete Muscle Release
*by Yamuna Zake and Stephanie Golden*

**The Heart of Yoga**
Developing a Personal Practice
*by T. K. V. Desikachar*

**The Five Tibetans**
Five Dynamic Exercises for Health, Energy, and Personal Power
*by Christopher S. Kilham*

**Like a Fish in Water**
Yoga for Children
*by Isabelle Koch*

**The Yoga-Sutra of Patañjali**
A New Translation and Commentary
*by Georg Feuerstein*

**Yoga for the Three Stages of Life**
Developing Your Practice As an Art Form, a Physical Therapy, and a Guiding Philosophy
*by Srivatsa Ramaswami*

**Inner Traditions • Bear & Company**
P.O. Box 388 • Rochester, VT 05767 • 1-800-246-8648
www.InnerTraditions.com

Or contact your local bookseller